Chimera

Chimera

Living Through Leukaemia

A Memoir

Jody White

Ω

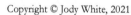

First published in the United Kingdom 2021
This edition published 2021 by Lumieres Press

www.lumierespress.com

A catalogue record for this book is available from the British Library

ISBN: PB: 978-1-7399612-0-6; eBook: 978-1-7399612-1-3;
Audiobook: 978-1-7399612-2-0

Typeset by Jody White
Printed in the UK

Also available as an eBook and Audiobook

To find out more about Jody, please visit www.jodywhite.co.uk

For my family and for Tasha

CONTENTS

Author's Note   i-ii
Omega   iii-iv
Prologue   1

PART 1: SENTIENCE

1   The First Cut   9
2   Diagnosis Day   26
3   Admittance   41
4   Red Sky At Night   51
5   Lumbar Puncture   64
6   Operation Cell Death   78

PART 2: INITIATION

Ω   The Cowboy   91
7   The Gospel of Leuk   96
Ω   Time is Tight   115
8   Freedom   120

Ω	Angus & Kelly	133
9	I See You	137
Ω	Target Secured	152
10	Morphine Dreams	157
Ω	Innerspace	170
11	Back To Reality	173
Ω	The Dark Moon	193
12	Transplant	196

PART 3: SOLVE ET COAGULA

Ω	The Bone Collector	211
13	Shifting Seasons	213
Ω	The Hunt	227
14	My Sister's Bones	229
Ω	Fire Made Flesh	242
15	Prisoner	244
Ω	Sounding Body	255
16	Moments of Clarity	257
Ω	Wolfboy	268
17	Adulting	270

Epilogue	287
Acknowledgements	299
Supporting Chimera	302
Crowdfunder Supporters	303
About the Author	306
Blood and Marrow	308

Author's Note

It struck me what it means to live with a myth, and
what it means to live without one (...) so, in the most
natural way, I took it upon myself to get to know
my myth, and this I regarded as my task of tasks.

Carl Jung

I have come to understand the telling of this story, the tale of my
life-threatening illness, as a way to explore my personal mythology.
Our lives are composed of stories. Ones you might tell freely to
those around you or ones you keep to yourself, hidden away inside
your heart. The concept is simple: key periods of life can become
stories in and of themselves, separate from their protagonists, *if* we
are courageous enough to share them.

You are about to read the defining story of my life so far. It
invokes the archetypal hero's journey as seen through the extremely
personal experience of acute disease. The crystallisation of wisdom
can begin under the greatest of pressures. Through sharing our

stories, especially those of challenge or difficulty, I believe it is possible that their leaden weight can be more deeply understood; their potential to transform us unlocked, as they undergo a final transmutation into pieces of pure gold. That is the work of true personal alchemy.

It is my wish that this book can help bring some form of hope to anyone dealing with a life-threatening diagnosis. I offer my thoughts to those recently diagnosed or currently undergoing any form of treatment, whether you're in or out of the hospital, GPs' surgeries and specialist clinics – whatever your prognosis. I would like to extend these sentiments to all the family and friends who, it is important to remember, intently feel the impact of such diagnoses upon their kin. Stay strong for yourself and for those around you, but know that there is no shame in crying, nothing wrong with really expressing and embodying your feelings, however negative you, or society, might deem them.

For those of you blessed to have never been in such a position, I would counsel you to cultivate a daily sense of gratitude for all you have, all that feeds your life, however small and simple those things appear to be. May you open your heart to the reality of those around you who are currently suffering, or who have suffered – there are many of us around. It could be the elderly lady you sat next to on the bus to work this morning, the bright-eyed young man who made your coffee, or the rosy-cheeked child who giggled when you pulled a silly face at her in the street.

Ω

Omega

As you move through this book, you will come across the use of the Omega. This potent symbol is deeply intertwined with many fundamental aspects of human life, even down to its use denoting the year or date of a person's death.

Once known primarily as the 24th and last letter of the ancient Greek alphabet, today the Omega is utilised across a variety of different contexts and disciplines. You may have seen it appear in the company branding of a famous watch manufacturer, or as the logo of popular video game *God of War*.

Christianity also uses it, along with the first letter, Alpha. The Book of Revelation famously describes God as 'the Alpha and the Omega', generally translated as the beginning and end of all things. Another way to think of this is as *eternity*: that place of dreamy timelessness that exists beyond the boundaries of life.

In astrology, there exist the *lunar nodes*, two points where the moon crosses the ecliptic whilst on its orbit around the Earth. There is an ascendant node and descendant node. The ascending node, commonly known as the North Node, is symbolised by the Omega. The South, or descending node, is the Omega inverted. It was used to predict eclipses, since they only occurred close to the nodes. It is also has a strong association with the twelfth and final sign of the Zodiac, Pisces.

As a counterbalance to its deep mythic and spiritual roots, the Omega is widely used by the sciences. In chemistry it represents the stable natural oxygen isotope, oxygen-18. In physics it is the *ohm*, a unit of electrical resistance, while in astronomy it represents the density of the universe. It is also used in the fields of mathematics, genomics, computer science and statistical mechanics.

In molecular biology, the symbol is used as shorthand to signify a genetic construct introduced by a *two-point crossover*: a recombination of differing genetic information to create new offspring.

Clearly, there exists time-honoured symbolism for the Omega to denote the ending of great cycles. A universal representation of death, destruction and change.

Prologue

What is a myth? It's a framework or a story drawn from aspects of the psyche or society. Because myths contain truths which we can all recognise, it's human nature to project our own life experiences onto them. In doing so, we start to make sense of our lives and the things that have happened to us.

Thinking about our life's journey in terms of myth and story helps us to understand the various roles we may have been playing, and can bestow a unique level of awareness to our patterns of behaviour. This in turn allows us to make conscious changes when we are able.

The *hero's journey* is a famous mythic framework often applied to peak human experiences. This so-called monomyth, or myth of all myths, popularised by Joseph Campbell's book *The Hero With A Thousand Faces*, details a core structure that has informed the plots of countless books, films, and legends throughout recent history. It goes a little something like this: the hero decides to embark upon a quest, faces a series of challenges along the way, yet ultimately returns to share the tale of his/her success with those they left behind. It's a classic trope.

The mythology of the hero's journey is especially evident in the context of a human being faced with a life-threatening illness. Such experiences are commonly framed as battles to be fought and therefore, something either won or lost. The prize being a celebrated victory over the ultimate enemy: death.

The use of metaphor or myth to make sense of life is unavoidable for us humans. This is because we live within the universe of a collective mythology; layers of metaphor underpin all that we do. We cannot escape them. In the context of myth, the experience of a life-threatening diagnosis is closely aligned with an underworld journey.

In this scenario, the protagonist is simply going about their life when the ground beneath their feet gives way and they are swept into a strange new world where all the rules have been flipped upside down and nothing is quite what it seems. This descent, or katabasis as the Ancient Greeks would say, also forms an integral part of the hero's journey. In this process the self is broken apart and dissolved. Within the chaos that follows, the protagonist has the opportunity to re-assemble themselves into a whole new form.

Alchemy is often associated with slightly unhinged 12th century scientists and their attempts to transmute base metals into gold. This, however, is somewhat of a distracting metaphor. For centuries, esoteric philosophers have used alchemy as a complex spiritual framework, its ultimate goal being personal transformation. The aim here is for *us* to become the gold, as we attempt to live up to our highest potential. The first stage is known as calcination. In this stage, the raw material is broken down into its constituent parts so that it may be re-formed anew. *Solve and Coagula* – dissolve and re-form – are key alchemical principles and calcination can therefore be understood as the first stage in a potent process of spiritual rebirth.

Adopting mythology as a cancer survival strategy was instinctive. Back then, lying in my hospital room on the night I was admitted, a conscious decision was made to confront the diseased parts of myself, whilst working to accept the possibility of death. Wielding what little choice I did have, I decided to make these rogue cells and their wayward biological processes my enemies. I knew that deep down I wasn't ready to die. I was young, fit, and eager to seek the opportunities and experiences life could offer. Exciting things had only just started to happen. At the threshold of adulthood, an independent life was yet to fully begin and I was determined not to miss it.

As a cancer patient, this applied version of the hero's journey, where death itself becomes the enemy, is one thrust upon you by society. The cultural and social expectation was to fight. The patient is expected to follow the framework of the story by embarking on the quest for life and engaging in the ensuing battle. As heroes go, the cancer patient is somewhat passive. This journey is forced upon them. They are even likely to be celebrated for the suffering they undergo and those around them may bestow them with special status.

Some patients find this extremely useful. It can help provide the courage and strength of a brave warrior in an attempt to will the body into healing, to rid it of diseased cells, and eventually return to full health. Of course, there are no guarantees, and some would say adopting such an approach sets the patient and their loved ones up for further grief and mental anguish should this journey end in death rather than some kind of 'heroic' victory.

Others may feel the pressure to put up a fight immensely overwhelming at a time when all their energy is being sapped. It takes all they have just to get themselves out of bed each morning. They might prefer there was no fight, no battle, simply a living awareness that the body has been given a medical diagnosis and their only job is to be present with it, open to any outcome. I appreciate this standpoint because it doesn't personify the disease as negative, it accepts cancer for what it is: a set of confused biological processes.

The rare few may eventually choose to fully accept their death. Choosing to die is still very much a cultural taboo, but ultimately, it is the individual's sovereign right to make those decisions. It can be for no-one else to judge.

Crucially, the question I held was not *what am I fighting against?* Fighting against my own body, effectively fighting against death, was simply not going to work. This felt like a denial. It did not come from a place of fierce love. I was forced to acknowledge my death very early on. I had to be realistic. I knew that the cancer cells might ultimately be too great in number to be overcome. Any warrior headed into the unknown understands that they may not return, yet my desire to stay alive was unshakeable.

In my case, the key question was very clearly *what am I fighting for?* I knew that I loved my family and my girlfriend. I wanted to fight for their love, for a chance at a future with them. I wanted to fight because I loved myself and felt deeply that this disease did not belong in my life. And if, despite it all, I were to die anyway, why not go out giving it everything I had? At least I could say that I fought in the name of love. I count myself lucky to have had something tremendous worth fighting for.

With that said, I feel it is important to mark a show of force, the defence of one's boundaries, as distinct from more overt military metaphors. Not all force denotes a war. It can be an innately self-protective mechanism, much as an Aikido master would take the approaching energy of his opponent and divert it so as to use it against them. The defence of all I held dear felt appropriate, necessary. After all, at the cellular level an incredible battle *was* occurring – the foot-soldiers and assassins of my immune system were furiously engaged every second of every day. My body was fighting to return to *homeostasis*, the place of balance where all of our systems are functioning efficiently. When attempting to harness the eliminatory power of the immune system, I believe it makes sense to think and act as it does. Without being fully aware of it at the time, this is what I tried to do.

Part One

SENTIENCE

To go in the dark with a light is to know the light.
To know the dark, go dark. Go without sight,
and find that the dark, too, blooms and sings,
and is travelled by dark feet and dark wings.

Wendell Berry

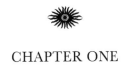

CHAPTER ONE

The First Cut

Sometimes, life has a way of breaking us apart and dissolving the roots of who we thought we were, before slowly piecing us back together anew.

In 1999, I was a shy and sensitive seventeen-year-old with only a single and a rather brief relationship to my name. After years of pubescent angst, I was excited to finally experience this new form of connection.

Tamsin was sexy and aloof and I constantly felt like I was dreaming while I was with her, walking on air because *she had chosen me*. We'd wander around Bridgnorth's High Town together, looking in shop windows and kissing under the spring blossoms in Castle Park. Like so many before us, we'd hold hands in the back row of the local indie cinema, pausing at her doorstep on the way home.

To help express my torrent of feelings, I'd played her a track from a *Q Magazine* compilation – 'Saint' by Texas – in which Sharleen Spiteri pledges her entire life to her beloved.

She dumped me after a few short weeks.

When pressed for a reason, her response was that I was just 'too nice'. Clearly, this fledgling take on romance had not worked in my favour. I was hurt and frustrated. Did that mean she wanted me to care less?

Relationships aside, I'd done well to navigate the social strata on my journey through Bridgnorth Endowed School. I got along well with the football lads, the computer geeks, the shy girls, the it-girls, the awkward kids shuttled in from small surrounding villages, the laid-back music lovers, and the more open-minded teachers. I adored anyone who could adopt the role of class comedian.

The popular girls laughed at my sardonic humour and we'd hang out, but I was careful never to get too close. Instead, I admired them from afar, dreaming up elaborate, hormonally-charged fantasies in which they starred. I hadn't the first clue about the art of seduction or how to handle the complexities of the opposite sex. Firmly in my favour were my well-honed skills behind a drum kit which had proved to be a real asset when it came to attracting attention.

Our band went by the terrible name of Identical Footwear, so-called because we all wore Kickers, the brand of choice for teenage males in the late 1990s. Rob, Rishi, Pete, and I would spend our lunch hours jamming away in the school's music room. This display of youthful creativity began to attract a small crowd of our peers to the tall glass windows which lined three sides of the space. They'd crane their necks to get a better view as we cranked out surprisingly decent versions of Led Zeppelin's 'Rock N' Roll' and

Smashing Pumpkin's 'Zero'. Not bad for a bunch of fresh-faced lads who could barely grow a bumfluff moustache, despite an uncanny ability to get served lukewarm pints of lager in the Carpenters Arms on any given Friday night.

Tasha hung around in the crowd who came to watch our band practices. We'd locked eyes briefly a couple of times. I had always been quietly fascinated by her but could count the times we'd actually spoken to each other on the fingers of one hand. She was friends with the in-crowd but she wasn't really one of them. While they revelled in their premium status amongst the social hierarchy, she presented a smiling old soul that oozed kindness and a wild, barely hidden sexuality that signalled heaven to me. I thought she was perfect. Her tumbling, dirty-blonde bob had a life of its own, while experience shone from her sharp blue eyes. A streetwise tone coloured her edges as if she carried with her the weight of a secret burden. I wondered what it was.

She sat on the back row of GCSE geography, chatty and bright, charming the male teachers with her sweet maturity, equally as bolshy as the lads. Some people have a certain air about them, an invisible energy that draws others in. She was like that. Sexy, but not conventionally so. Feminine, yet tomboyish with her paint-splattered jeans and rusty-red Camper shoes. She was completely genuine and wore her heart firmly on her sleeve, a combination so unusual in this environment and consequently extremely alluring.

I willed courage into my body almost daily to gain the strength to talk to her and to look into those glassy blue eyes for just a few long seconds. I wanted to soak myself in that delicious tingle that snaked itself around my chest whenever she was around. It was no good just staring at her and then trying to hide it if she so much as raised her head in my direction. If it was a particularly good day I might even try projecting my feelings to her telepathically in an attempt to make her understand.

Finally, I realised I needed a little help. My friend Jamie took A-level Art. Tasha was in the same class and I knew they hung out together, smoked straights outside the school gates at four o'clock, and were both generally on board with the classic tenets of teen rebellion. Jamie was something of a wild card with a difficult home-life. He could be unpredictably mean yet it was clear age was making him kinder to those he actually liked. I approached him on the way out of last period, at the corner of the school where sweaty locker rooms met bleached-clean toilets, and the solemnity of the Maths department lay just beyond the threshold double doors.

'Hey dude.'

'Oh hey Jode, how it going?'

'Yeah good, good. Just wondering if you could do me a favour–' I began. He shot me a quizzical grin.

'Yeah, of course, mate.'

'Cool, it's just, umm, well… Tasha… you know her right?'

'Yeah, Tash is cool. Do you like her then or something?'

'Well, yeah, I do and I just thought, maybe, you could mention me to her?'

It was a relief to actually say it. I felt as if I was opening some kind of door to the future.

'Ask her if she likes me, if she wants to go out with me… I'd really appreciate it.'

'Haha, interesting… Yeah, she's a really sound girl. Actually, I think she split up with someone not long ago, but I'll see what I can do. We've got art tomorrow morning so she should be there.'

'Thanks mate, I really appreciate it. Catch you later.'

'Yeah, sure loverboy. Laters.' He smirked.

The Klixx vending machine clicked and whirred, making me a watery coffee. It was almost 9.30 am and most people had drifted off to class. Jamie arrived to report his dramatic findings: Tasha was into me too. I knew this was my chance to act, step up, and be the man who took a risk in the name of love, or whatever you might call this bizarre feeling. My heart began to pump faster, flushing my cheeks. I was scared shitless at the thought of seeing her armed with this new information.

Minutes later, as I was about to leave the building, already late for English, and knelt down trying to stuff my jacket into a bursting backpack, I saw her. Tasha was walking up the stairs at the far end of the corridor. She was dressed in a short-sleeved checkered shirt that hugged her curves, her baggy blue boot-cuts sashayed this way and that, while round-toed scarlet shoes poked out playfully from beneath them.

She would have to pass me. We would have to speak. Oh fuck.

I panicked, almost balked, almost said nothing. I fumbled nervously with the zip on my bag. Just as she was about to draw level, her eyes flashed to mine.

'Hey,' I blurted.

'Hi.'

'Can I talk to you?'

'Sure.' She smiled, a flush of pink in her cheeks. A faint smell of cigarette smoke.

Can I talk to you? I cursed my linguistic shyness. *What the fuck sort of a line is that? What an idiot.* For a minute or two, we skirted around the obvious, talked about friends and school, and then—

'So did Jamie mention anything the other day…?' I asked.

A long pause.

'Yeah, he did. I'm flattered, I… I don't know what to say.'

She doesn't like me, she thinks I'm an idiot. Say something.

'I've kind of just split up with someone and I'm not ready to start anything else just yet.'

Shit. Fuck. Darkest of black days, torrential apocalyptic thunderstorms, a whirlpool of epic proportions sucking me DOWN DOWN DOWN…

'But we should hang out sometime. How about Friday night, you going to be out?'

Sweet Jesus, I'm saved.

'Yeah, I should be around. Everyone going to the Castle as usual?'

'I should think so. Me, Anna and Laura will be there. You should come along, it'll be fun.'

That sideways smile, those dazzling eyes.

'Ok cool. I will.' Could she hear the sound of my heart thumping in my throat?

Months of yearning, praying and attempted telepathy had somehow paid off. The girl I wanted was within my reach. It was July and the nights were long and warm. Fridays were the highlight of the social calendar in Bridgnorth. The route between pubs would develop organically over the course of an evening, with arrangements and rendezvous points quickly spread through a new technology called the text message.

The Old Castle was ramshackle in the classic English style, replete with an ageing jukebox, fruit machines aplenty and a knackered pool table in a room of its own out back, its luminous green felt dotted with small rips and the odd fag burn. The too-old-to-still-be-drinking propped up the bar while the too-young-to-drink gathered for the first few rounds before the next establishment was decided and the herd gradually moved on. Pints, shots, alco-pops. Tipple after tipple. I wasn't much of a drinker. I'd have a few too many if it was the right sort of night; the ones where you can feel friendships being forged and where boundaries melt away, but I knew my limits and didn't enjoy obliterating my brain cells anywhere near as much as everyone else.

This particular night, however, called for a special effort. I took a long shower, fastidiously cleaning and lathering every limb and crevice then swilling off the bubbles with the steaming hot water. I spent time blow-drying my hair and applying dabs of hair putty. I even stole a few puffs of Mum's hairspray. Then I had to decide what to wear – *what would impress her?*

I was of medium-slim build, though I'd recently introduced a few eager sit-ups and push-ups to my morning routine. Following the progress of my muscles in the mirror satisfied my unfolding teenage ego. I swiped a small bottle of Belgian lager from the fridge and sat in my room listening to Rage Against The Machine, the furious music imparting a sense of purpose, priming my confidence for the evening ahead.

I checked my Nokia, no new texts. As was traditional, I met my good friend Rob at the junction of Queensway Drive and Dunval Close and together we sauntered towards the bustling town centre where over a dozen pubs lay within a few minutes' walk of each other. After getting our pints at The Castle's main bar, we moved past the old-timers to the terraced garden where all the kids hung out. Immediately, I saw her. Tasha was sat at a picnic bench drinking a White Russian, shining like a beacon in a tight white shirt.

That night was dreamlike, rare in its lucidity. As the laughter rang out and the drinks flowed we exchanged lingering looks, flirting with the tension, territory marked out by the closeness of our bodies. Hours flew by. Things became fluid, softly blurred at the edges. My confidence soared.

The group mind shifted and the next location was decided. The Carpenter's Arms was a small and lively pub on the other side of town, a particular favourite amongst those who straddled the boundary of the UK's legal drinking age. Tasha and I pitched up at the bar, leaning over the towelled mats and stainless steel drip trays to make an order. Jack Daniels and Coke was the drink for this point in the evening, the sweet, black elixir with a kick in the tail. Laura ordered Bacardi Breezers, nudging me in the ribs with a less-than-subtle wink, and we all sat down around a small wooden table. Just me and three lovely young ladies. I felt like a king.

Tash caught my eye. 'You ok?'

'I am definitely ok,' I replied, grinning.

'Well that's good.' She kissed my cheek, leapt up, and shimmied her way over to the jukebox, put on some Stone Roses, and danced her way off to the toilets.

As she sat back down, I took a deep breath. It was time for a little boldness. Under the table, my right hand slipped smoothly onto Tasha's left thigh. She smiled but continued her conversation across the table with Laura. Then, taking a sip of her drink, she responded with a reciprocal manoeuvre, her eyes flicking to meet mine.

After this daring first move, things went better than I could have hoped. Leaving the pub, we walked the length of the High Street hand in hand, tipsy and giggling, not caring who saw us. An indie-disco was held every other Friday above the Comrades Club in a large wooden-floored room. You could drink until 1 am, so we all flocked there after last orders at the pubs.

Inhibitions truly dissolved, we hit the dance-floor, holding each other close, snaking in time to the beat and the pulse. Beneath the smoke, flashing deep reds and greens lit up our bodies. The rest of the room fell away, only her eyes remained in sharp focus. Suddenly I kissed her and all at once she became mine. Our mouths pressed together, all soft lips and trembling tongues. Perfume. Cigarettes. Sweat. The testosterone flowed. I lost all track of time.

At 2 am, the staff began kicking us all out.

'I've got to go now Jode, but I've had such a great night.'

'Me too Tash, when can I see you again?' I was breathless, hungry for more.

'I'm going away for a few weeks over the summer, all the girls are going to Tenerife and then I'm going to Africa with my family. But I'll send you a postcard, let's swap addresses,' she instructed, handing me a piece of tattered blue paper and a pen from her bag.

Details duly imparted, we withdrew to the main doorway, where we hugged and softly kissed again. Then she was gone, her smell on my t-shirt and the watery, indescribable taste of her on my tongue. I was dazed and drunk. It was long gone two and sleep beckoned. I decided to walk home, still not quite able to take it all in. What strange magic was this? This smart, sassy girl was truly into me. I felt invincible which worked wonders for my wavering self-esteem. For a brief while, life felt perfect.

Summer bloomed into lazy days with nowhere to be and nothing to do, a time that seems to exist only in the haze of teenage memories. We barely saw each other, though every couple of weeks, a cute illustrated postcard would arrive with details of where she'd been and what she'd been up to. The first one had a garish Tenerife sunset slapped on the front and a message scrawled in thick red pen over most of the reverse, with absolutely no concern for the neat four lines of allotted space. I pictured her bumming a pen from some helpless shopkeeper:

Hey you !
Having a great time in Tenerife, all the girls say hi.
See you soon, miss you,
T xx

I spent much of my time daydreaming about her. I'd ride my bike down through the suburbs of the town, across the river and along to Severn Park, following the path along the riverside to the wildflower meadows at the far end, the part where they didn't cut the grass as often and where no-one really went.

My backpack contained a bottle of water, my smoking tin, and a selection of books. Half stuck to the inside pocket was the remains of a sticky bag of boiled sweets. I'd sit by the river, plugged into my music player, a battered notepad close at hand. I wrote poems, diary entries, all my wishes and fears, thoughts, and impressions. It was as if some dormant cognitive function in my brain was now fully active. I felt renewed and inspired, completely buzzing with vital life force energy.

In Ibiza, my family had rented a small villa on the outskirts of Santa Eularia. We baked our bodies on and off for almost two weeks in the Balearic heat. I spent the days lying on the terracotta tiled roof, gazing up at the endless blue sky, then wandering down to the beach in the afternoons to cool off in the glassy Mediterranean.

I devoured a couple of Russell Hoban books. My parents laughed a lot and got mildly sunburnt. My two younger sisters, Jemma and Jessie, dunked each other in the pool, while my little brother Josh watched, grinning from ear to ear, before boldly taking a running jump into the water himself. We ate freshly baked baguettes smothered in thick garlic aioli, ordered steaming paella, and sipped bottles of chilled San Miguel.

In the darkness of my bedroom, wrapped in a sun-kissed glow, I envisioned Tasha lying next to me. As I fell asleep, I tried to calculate the distance that lay between us. Where was she? Who was she with? Was she thinking of me too?

As we took our last trips around the island, I became aware that such thoughts were being slowly replaced by a creeping sense of paranoia. We'd be in the car driving back from lunch on the beach or a walk around a small fishing village and a sudden feeling of dread would descend upon me. My bountiful happiness wavered. The rash that had been appearing on and off since we arrived had finally decided to hang around and make itself noticed. All across my stomach and spreading around to my back was a raised area of pinky-red skin that itched like hell. It had spread along the inside of my left thigh too and any amount of cream wouldn't persuade it to leave. My muttering and complaining was starting to affect the general mood.

'Calm down, you've probably just overdone the sun a little,' Dad said matter-of-factly. From the kitchen, Mum shouted something about making sure I was using Factor 30.

'Give it until we get home, I'm sure it'll have gone by then love… and listen to your mother.' His confident smile eased my worries. He turned back to his book, a chunky Len Deighton, took a sip of his beer, and adjusted the position of his faded baseball cap. I believed him. Parents have a knack for knowing just what to say to sooth their offspring's frazzled edges.

Monday the 6th of September. The first day of the rest of my life. Our first days as A-level students. We'd graduated from secondary school and were now entering the twilight of our teenage years. We were losing our innocence, slowly maturing.

I had barely stopped thinking about Tasha all summer and

had worked myself up into a nervous wreck before breakfast. This was it. We would finally get to cement our relationship and make it real. I knew she felt the same. She had to. She knew they were no ordinary kisses, it was not just another Friday night out on the town. We had started something there, under the flickering strobe lights.

At 8.55 am Mr. Phelps, the head of sixth-form, ambled into the common room from his adjoining office. 'Alright you philistines… shut up, shut up!' boomed his deep Welsh accent. A few titters bounced around the room but no one wanted to make a fuss on the first day back so we gamely took our seats for the register. She still wasn't here. My heart was pounding. I tried to ignore it.

'Matthews…'

'Here sir.'

'Miss Jones...'

'Sir.'

'Mr Davies...' he repeated.

A few sniggers leaked out.

'Mr Davies...?' he called once more. He paused to survey the room over the top of his thick black spectacles.

'If someone would be so kind as to suppress their giggles and inform me of the whereabouts of Mr Davies then I would be eternally grateful.'

'He's taking a dump sir,' someone said. More sniggers.

'Fantastic. Ahem, where was I…' He cleared his throat, ran his forefinger down the list.

He was about to continue when the double doors swung open and Tasha burst through, her skin tanned and smooth, her cheeks flushed. Turning, she picked me out of the crowd and flashed a quick smile, I thought I might crack.

'Sorry sir. We had a problem with the car on the way in.' She grinned and took a seat next to Anna.

'Thank you Miss Clode. Now, where were we…'

I became flushed and self-conscious and looked away, fiddled with my laces, slid my hand inside the front section of my backpack. I wrapped my fingers around the paper bag which contained the few small gifts I'd selected at the hippie market in Es Canar and gripped it like a trophy.

After registration people wandered out to the first lessons of the day. A few groups lingered, catching up on the gossip. Tasha was sat with two of her friends by a window that looked out over the faded concrete of the year 11 yard. I approached them, trying to look confident, trying to feel at ease. Anna noticed me first, then Laura with a knowing smile. Tash turned to me, her blue eyes sparkled. I thought I might turn to stone but somehow I managed to force out some words. Anna and Laura got up and left and suddenly there were just the two of us.

'Hey, you ok?' I started.

'It's been a weird morning Jode, but yes. All the better for seeing you,'

She gave me a big hug. My heart danced.

'How was your summer? I missed you.'

'I missed you too. Did you get my postcards?'

'Yeah, I loved them.'

'It was a funny summer. I'll tell you all about it later.'

'I brought you these…' I began, sifting through the contents of my backpack to find the market gifts.

I watched as she unwrapped the contents, praying I hadn't gone too far.

'Oh wow, I love them!' She blushed, smiling. 'Thank you.'

Tash planted a soft kiss on my burning cheek and looked right into me with those piercing blue eyes. At that moment, I decided I would do everything in my power to keep that look on her face.

As we walked, I slipped my hand into hers, her warm fingers gave a light squeeze in reply. Reaching the door where our paths divided, I moved to kiss her but before I could, she hugged me and said, 'Let's meet at free period.' She pecked me on the cheek and bounded away. I watched her go. As she reached the corner and was about to vanish, she turned back, flashed me a grin, and was gone.

Without really trying, we fell into a natural groove and spent much of the next few weeks together – kissing, talking into the early hours, getting tipsy on weak beer, and high on cheap hash. I lost my virginity to Tasha in the living room of my parent's house on their red and green floral sofa one late September afternoon when we should really have been at school. She had a little more experience than me, which helped my confidence. We got so carried away in the moment that at some point in the proceedings, I realised we hadn't even bothered to close the curtains. With my face pressed to her bare breast, a wave of embarrassment hit me.

'Tash, the curtains…'

Barely opening her eyes, she pulled me closer, and whispered into my ear, 'Leave them.'

By October, autumn had truly arrived, with its dramatic colour-ways and particular quality of light. The slowly bruising sky told me it was late afternoon and the school day was winding up. A bunch of us hung around in our usual common-room spot, the corner seats by the floor-to-ceiling window which commanded a general's-eye view over the playground. Laughing and joking and general piss-taking ensued, everyone participating in the comedy of the moment. The CD player pumped out the new Incubus album which held us in raptures. Tasha walked in. The double doors swung back and the rest of the world slowed to a crawl. I drank in the high dimples in her cheeks that shone when she laughed. She winked at me.

Jamie, sitting off to the right of the group, caught my eye. I felt the sweat start to form patches under my arms and tried to steady myself, leaning back from the chatter bubble. Tasha and her friend Hilda, a German exchange student, headed straight for the corner, taking their seats along the row of blue chairs with a volley of upbeat hellos and how's-it-goings, a quick kiss for me. A few strongly machined coffees and some cheap chocolate bars later, there were only the four of us left. Everyone else had classes to go to, cigarettes to smoke, or pubs to frequent. Jamie and I sat opposite the girls. Tash squeezed my feet while he practiced his flirtation techniques on the helpless Hilda. Eventually, Tasha and her friend left to catch their lift, and Jamie went off to his car.

After they'd all gone, I noticed a small piece of crumpled white paper on the seat where Tash had been sitting. I picked it up and unfolded it. It was a page ripped from her school workbook, over which were scrawled various games of squares and several love sums. Across one corner in blue biro were the words:

Tasha Clode loves Jody White

CHAPTER TWO

Diagnosis Day

Since returning to school, Tasha and I saw each other regularly. She lived with her family in a converted mill, tucked away at the bottom of a pretty dingle out in the Shropshire countryside. The house was picture-perfect, split over three levels with a brook running past the ample gardens. She'd laugh at my terrible jokes and we'd drink Red Stripe while Orbital's *In Sides* pulsed out from the CD player.

Lying on her bed, the girl with the sun in her head would trace her fingers along my forearm, triggering waves of sparks underneath my skin. Time ceased to be linear. We were merging into each other's worlds and life had taken on a whole new sparkle, despite the shortening days.

Thoughts of the past faded from my mind. I barely even dreamt of the future. She drew me into the now, that mysterious place where she lived. She helped me learn how to feel alive there, open to the birth of opportunity. That sense of excitement was intoxicating and her company quickly became a place I wanted to return to again and again.

Tempering this efflorescent love were various ailments that had been irritating me for some time. The mysterious rashes of the summer had abated; in their place were a variety of other anomalies: earaches, unexplained bouts of feeling run-down, and a tickly-dry throat that stubbornly refused to go away. Most recently, I had woken up one day in early October with the volume knob of my world turned down a few notches. Sounds were muffled and I struggled to hear what people were saying; clearly, I needed to get checked out.

Bridgnorth Medical Practice was situated in a tall townhouse on the High Street, fronted by an imposing red door. The waiting room was tucked away at the rear of the building inside an ornate Victorian conservatory filled with lush tropical plants and a trickling water feature. Unfortunately, these pretty facades were unable to mask the timeless weight of sickness. The unnatural stench of sanitiser hung like winter mist over the room as its motley crew of occupants waited to be prescribed their various pills and potions.

Each time I went to the surgery, the doctor would repeat the same procedure: a huge plastic thermometer would be inserted into my ear, then my blood pressure was taken with one of those ugly pump-up cuffs. Finally, he'd gaze down my throat, spying on my tonsils with his jet black pen-torch. I would leave with a prescription for penicillin, or a steroid cream, or some antibiotic ear-drops. Each time these things did nothing to fix my issues. The hearing loss was the real icing on the cake though. At this point I was acutely aware that something wasn't working properly in my skinny teenage body, and I was beginning to get depressed. Tasha and my family were understanding but they couldn't do much more than offer their hopeful reassurance that things would no doubt improve. My latest visit had proved no different.

'If these don't work then we'll have to do a blood test,' Doctor Goodall said. 'There's always a chance it could be glandular fever. It's quite common at your age.'

I wasn't sure if this was supposed to make me feel better and I left the surgery with gloom hanging off my face. I was walking up the High Street towards the iconic North Gate, heading for home, when I saw Tasha coming towards me, pulling a young girl along behind her.

'Hey!' She seemed half pleased, half-embarrassed to see me.

'Hey Tash,' I said and planted a quick kiss on her lips.

'Say hello Ches—'

'Hi Francesca.' I tried a smile and a wave. She frowned back at me, defiantly silent.

'What did they say?' asked Tash.

'He thinks it's some sort of virus. Couldn't be sure though. They gave me these,' I replied, I shook my green and white striped pharmacy bag with faux-triumph. 'It's so fucking annoying. It's been two weeks now and I still don't feel any better. I wish it would just all go away.'

'It'll be alright,' she said, laying her hand gently on top of my shoulder.

Francesca giggled. We ignored her.

'Wait and see if the new drugs do something. And if they don't… you can give them to me!' She laughed.

'Yeah right.' I rolled my eyes. 'Look, I've gotta get back for dinner, I'll see you tomorrow. Are we still on for *American Beauty* on Friday?'

'As long as we don't need to get you a hearing aid, Mister.' She poked my chest playfully.

I wrinkled my nose, flashing pretend daggers, and leant over to kiss her cheek. It blushed pink at the touch. The fine light hairs on her face smelled like coconut.

'See you later, Hot Stuff,' she said.

I turned and watched them wander off down the street hand in hand like two drunken pirates, laughing and bumping into each other, swaying to the invisible rhythms of the sea.

A week later at around half-past ten, I was sat in the third row of Ms. Mannion's A-level English language class, a sense of shame steadily glowing across my cheeks. My hearing was operating at about half its usual volume and consequently, I was having real trouble understanding what was being taught, enduring a rigorous piss-taking from my classmates as a result.

As the lesson progressed, I grew more and more frustrated. After class, I walked the short distance down the hill from the school grounds into town for yet another appointment. Enough was enough, something needed to be done. I saw a stand-in by the name of Doctor Allen, an amiable guy who I'd seen once before and immediately warmed to. He was happy to listen to what I had to say and appeared genuinely concerned with getting to the bottom of it all, quite refreshing given my previous experiences in the building.

'Ok Jody, I'm sorry that we haven't been able to find out what's causing your issues. I'm going to give you a prescription for some general antibiotics and book you in for a blood test at the hospital. They have a clinic open until 2 pm this afternoon so if you go down there now we should have the results back in a couple of days,' he informed. Then there was a pause. 'Alright?' He smiled awkwardly and handed me the freshly printed form.

I left the surgery with the folded paper clasped tightly in hand and wandered the short distance under the North Gate and down to the town's small general hospital. It was primetime for the lunch trade and the town centre was gently humming with local shoppers picking up their groceries and small gangs of kids sneaking out of school to buy a cone of chips.

I'd only been in the main hospital building once before, several years prior for a hernia operation. Memory served me up images of a dark, musty environment populated by people with drips and deep wrinkles, faces etched with sadness. It could have been the general anaesthetic but there was something strange about the way the shadows bounced around the bleached walls in that old brick building that made me feel like I'd walked onto the set of a low-budget arthouse horror film.

The blood clinic was situated around the back of the main complex in a newly built annexe. Its large glass windows let in plenty of natural light and subsequently felt much more comfortable. I announced myself to the middle-aged nurse on reception who crossed me off her list with practiced aplomb. Elderly warfarin patients read well-thumbed copies of *People's Friend* magazine and young children bawled after their booster injections. Everyone else looked ever-so-slightly nervous to be spending time in a place so steeped in the starkness of our own mortality.

They called me through after only a few minutes. The nurse had already done thirteen patients so far that morning and was in no mood for pleasantries. She sat next to me sternly, content with the stony silence. The tourniquet was tight and uncomfortable, my bulging veins wriggled like worms trapped under my skin. I turned to look out the window. I'd never had a blood test before. How simple it was, all over in a flash.

'Okay, now take a deep breath in please… sharp scratch.'

A rapid burning sensation flooded up my arm as she pierced the skin.

'Wow, that stung!'

'You've got very good veins,' she said, casually filling several vials of blood from a tube in the crook of my left arm.

'Err, thanks.'

The blood was surprisingly dark, like a fine Malbec. She labeled each tube and placed them into a tray.

'All done, you're free to go,' she got up and poked her head out the door.

'Next please.'

'Sorry, umm—do you know when I'll be able to find out the results?'

'We'll get them back to you tomorrow, just give your GP surgery a ring. Next please.'

Around 5 pm that same day, the phone in our hallway began to ring. Since the blood test, I'd been at home all afternoon, distracting myself from my rushing thoughts in any way I could, primarily by teasing my youngest sister Jessie and generally messing around. As I heard the shrill ringing echo through the house, part of me immediately knew the nature of the call, knew that my life was about to change. This knowing manifested as a torrent of anxiety that flew across my chest, spiralled up my spine, and finally paused to linger at the back of my heart. I couldn't bring myself to leave my bedroom and pick up the phone. I let it ring on.

While Dad was still at work in Wolverhampton and wouldn't be back until six, Mum had been working from her makeshift office on the wooden table in our dining room that afternoon. Jessie was on the sofa watching kid's TV.

I heard the handle creak as she opened the kitchen door and moved towards the bottom of the stairs. The ringing stopped. I sprang from my horizontal position on the bed and moved quietly to the top of the stairs, watching her from my elevated viewpoint, trying to gauge her reaction. She was listening and nodding. Saying, 'Of course... right... ok,' and then, 'we'll be down right away. Ok, thanks.'

Her face told a story I didn't want to hear, corroborating my fears. She realised I had been watching her and glanced up to the landing. I walked slowly down the carpeted stairs towards her. I could see her hazel eyes were beginning to water a little at the edges

'That was the doctors Jode, they've got your blood results back and they want to see us down at the surgery. They say it's quite important that we go as soon as we can.'

She was trying to hide her worry, trying so very hard.

'Did they say why?'

'No, just that we need to go down there now.'

'Oh God, Mum. It's going to be something horrible isn't it?' I said. Unease had turned to rising panic.

'Now we don't know that, let's just pop down and see what they have to say,' she replied. She turned away quickly to gather her jacket and car keys.

We left eleven-year-old Jessie on the sofa, her face quietly concerned, and climbed into Mum's tiny Nissan Micra. Neither of us said much on the short drive down into town until Mum broke the silence.

'It's probably just nothing, maybe a virus. Don't worry, it'll be ok.'

I don't think she really believed that but I appreciated the sentiment. Another wave of foreboding hit me, clearly, this was serious. I'm sure we both knew it, but neither of us wanted to feed the fear demons any bloody morsels.

Spotting a rare parking space on the High Street, we pulled up directly outside the surgery's front door. No hanging around in stuffy waiting rooms for us today, oh no. We were ushered in and straight up to the first floor where the doctors' rooms were located. After a couple of polite knocks, we were called into the plush wood-panelled office of one of the main partners. A rather slick and aloof man, I'd always felt repelled by his sour demeanour. What twisted irony then that he should be the one to deliver the news. I eyed him suspiciously as he began to speak a few words of greeting. He looked decidedly uncomfortable which was less than reassuring.

'Jody we received a call from the hospital an hour ago regarding your blood test. Your white blood cell count is three-hundred and twenty-three, that's extremely high. I'm afraid...' – he paused, perhaps trying to find the words – 'you have leukaemia.'

What can you say to that? What is the official reaction to a cancer diagnosis? Tears? Anger? Anguish? All of that. Yet at first, for me, there was simply nothing. A void.

For a second or two, my mind stuttered to a halt as if struck by a processing error, a neuronal collision. The past and future combined and contracted at lightspeed, slamming me into the distorted, twisted present. Life as I knew it collapsed, crumbled into dust, and fell through my fingers. School. My family. My girlfriend. My friends. Would I even live to see another week? I felt a throbbing headache coming on. Surely life couldn't be ending now, just as it was starting to truly begin? Something cracked inside me, as at my side, Mum uttered a guttural cry, crumpling into herself. I reached out for her hand and we gripped each other too tightly. We sat sobbing together, high on uncertainty, faced with the very real threat of an untimely and painful separation. I pressed my face into her woven woollen jacket, my tears and saliva pooling into a cocktail of dark stains.

'We'll fight this, we can fight this,' came her high-pitched whisper into my mess of hair.

I had no words with which to reply. She tried to pull herself together, using all of her strength to retain some degree of composure. I understood she was desperately trying to be strong for my sake. She asked the doctor a question as I zoned out, dazed and reeling, trying to catch my stuttering breath. Their voices became a blur of sound in the background. I felt the floor open up beneath me, its depth felt endless.

After what felt like forever, I wiped my eyes with Mum's tissues, blew my snotty nose, and looked up at the doctor. He shifted uncomfortably in his seat, his pale face painted with sorrow. He sighed deeply and looked down at his computer screen, searching for something helpful to say.

'Am I going to die?' I said.

A blank face. Bastard. He had no fucking idea.

'Well… There are many good treatments these days. There's every reason to have hope. There were a pair of young twins diagnosed in the town last year who are doing very well now. I can't say much more as it's not my field but we've been in touch with the Haematology Unit over at the Royal Shrewsbury Hospital. They've prepared a room and they'd like you in today.'

'What, right now?'

'Yes. They said it's critical that they start treatment and run further tests as soon as possible. Go home and get a bag together, some clothes and whatever else you need, then make your way there. They will be expecting you. I'm sorry to have to be the one to break this news,' he said. He seemed genuinely apologetic now, yet clearly uncomfortable to be sharing his office with this tsunami of raw emotion.

I felt something inside me clunking onwards, like the wheel of a giant metal cog turning. 'Ok. Well, let's get on with it then.'

Somehow we made it out of that suffocating panelled room and back outside to our little red car. A gaggle of spotty school kids shuffled past on their way home, shirts hanging out, laughing and joking. They have no idea of what just happened, I thought. They have no idea how precious their life is. We all take the gift of our aliveness for granted.

Mum drove numbly up through town, navigating Friday's post-work traffic up to the family home. Shattered and dazed, our entrance burst a bubble of teatime energy composed of my three younger siblings, the kitchen radio pumping out Radio 4's *Six O'Clock News* and Dad in the centre at the counter, a tea-towel slung across his shoulder, poised with his knife, chopping up vegetables for dinner. He took one look at our faces, dropped the knife, and ran towards the door.

'He's got leukaemia,' Mum blurted out, sobbing.

We folded into his arms in tears while my brother and sisters came to sit awkwardly around the kitchen table, unsure of how to react. I hugged them fiercely in turn until they too began to well up with tears.

As softly as she could through her evident pain, Mum tried to explain what the doctor had said. It was deadly serious. Her son, their brother, was very, very ill. I felt like she was talking about someone else, someone who wasn't sat right next to her holding her hand. But this was happening to me. I felt sick at the thought of what was going on inside my body. My bone marrow had gone rogue and turned against me, pumping out traitorous white blood cells and sending them off to cause havoc.

We sat together as dark clouds of uncertainty and loss loomed heavily above us. Everything was happening so fast and none of us knew anything about it other than the fact that my life depended on being admitted into the hospital that evening.

Dad went to the shops and brought me back a bag of snacks, usually tightly controlled in our house. Now it was different, suddenly I could have whatever I wanted. I went upstairs and limply began to pack a bag with some essentials. After throwing a few pairs of pants and favoured t-shirts into a pile, I slumped down to the floor with my back to the white radiator in the corner of the room. A fierce heat emanated from its core and I could feel its ridges begin to sear themselves into my skin through my shirt. I accepted the pain, willing it to make me feel something other than this.

The telephone that lived in our hallway was grey and old. Time-squashed particles of dust had morphed together to become faintly inlaid in the cracks around its base. I walked back to my room, cradling it with care, hoping it could support me as I made the call. I swallowed hard, my throat growing dry. I felt my leg muscles contracting. It'd been a matter of hours and I didn't feel ready to even talk about it, let alone think about what it could mean or where it might take me.

Nothing felt real, as if I'd slipped into a vivid and ludicrous nightmare with no way of waking myself up. I sat on the edge of my bed in my box-like bedroom and stared at the cheap plastic handset. That phone call remains the most heart wrenching I have ever had to make. The phone felt wrong to be lying in my hands. I just wanted to hold her body tightly, to hear her tell me everything would be alright.

Eventually, through several deep and quivering breaths, I dialled her number, halfway through realising I'd missed out a two. I wiped the wetness from my red and puffy eyes, re-dialled and held the phone close to my ear, leaning forward over the side of the bed. My eyes met the wooden floor and blinked a few times at the shrill ringing. Silence. Buzz. Silence. Buzz. Silence.

'Hello, this is Simon Clode,' a voice said curtly.

'Is Tasha there please, it's Jody,' I managed to mumble.

'Oh right, hello. Yes, she is, I'll just go and get her.'

There was a rattle as the phone was dropped, followed by a series of muffled bangs.

'Tasha! Telephone for you, it's Jody… Tasha! Did you hear me?!'

'Yes Dad, I'm fucking coming! Chill out.'

I braced myself.

'Hey you.'

'Hi Tash, how are you?'

'I'm good Jode, what's up, you sound down?'

'Well that's 'cause I am a bit down,' I choked.

'Oh Jody! What is it, tell me?'

'Where are you?'

'In the kitchen, why?'

'I think you should go up to your room, I'd like to talk to you there.'

'Okay, give me a second.'

I listened in as she crossed the warm kitchen floor and pictured her jogging up the thickly-carpeted stairs, pushing back her bedroom door, plastered with photos, and eventually landing with a flop on the soft blue double bed.

'I'm here, all ears. What's going on?'

'Well, you know my blood test today?'

'Yeah, was it all okay? Was it glandular fever like they thought?'

'Well, no. It wasn't okay Tash. It wasn't okay at all.'

Now the tears came. The bastards have a mean sense of timing. Tasha was quiet, she knew something bad was coming. This stopped her from speaking and gave me the space to compose myself.

'They… they found that my white-blood cell count was really

high. Like off the charts. I've been diagnosed with leukaemia...' I trailed off into muffled sobs as more tears tracked down my face. That set her off and she started to cry down the phone into my better ear. There we were, tucked away in our bedrooms several miles apart, both in floods of tears. Life had shattered. I felt a part of myself float up and out of my body to watch the scene unfold.

'Leukaemia... what? Like cancer? Oh fuck, Jode. What does that mean?' she asked. Her voice quivered slightly as my heart thumped.

'I'm not going to fucking die, Tash!' I surprised myself with the ferocity of my statement.

A silence emerged.

'I don't know what to say, I'm so sorry, Jody. You're going to be okay though, right?' she questioned. Her words were coming quicker, she sounded panicked.

'I don't know, Tasha. I just don't know. I've got to go into Shrewsbury hospital tonight, we're leaving in a few minutes. The doctor said they want to start treatment as soon as they can. They say because I'm young I have a good chance,' I explained. Did I really believe any of that? 'This can't be happening, it's not fair. It's not fucking fair!'

'I know Jode, I know. But you'll get through this. We'll get through this. I wish I could be there with you right now.'

We exchanged bruised farewell sentiments, devoid of their usual spark. I promised her I'd find out a number she could call for updates and she promised to come and see me the next day. I asked her not to tell anyone we knew, it was too soon for explanations.

What an ugly duty – to shatter our bright new love and infuse it with the scent of imminent death. I hung up the phone blurry-eyed and broken. I just wanted to climb into bed and wrap myself up in the duvet until it all went away.

A mixture of rage and fear brewed up inside me. I could almost sense the arrival of the vultures, watching the scene, riding high on the thermals. I wondered how long I had left in this world. At seventeen this is not the kind of question you expect to have to ask yourself. Nothing can prepare you, nothing can be taught. You can only take it as it hits you, feel the fullness of the blow, allow yourself to spin and fall. And then, somehow, summon the will to get back up again.

I had to gather a bag together. How do you pack for the indefinite? All I could do was focus on what was right in front of me: my battered holdall, a week's worth of underpants, a few clothes, and a toothbrush. Outside my window, the day had de-saturated to monochrome and lifeless tones of grey as the sun bid us goodnight. Dad came upstairs and gently knocked on my bedroom door.

'Come on, Jode,' he said softly. 'We'd better get going.'

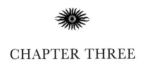

CHAPTER THREE

Admittance

It was almost dark when we left the house – Mum, Dad and I in the car. Temporary roadworks and the obligatory tractor held up traffic for part of the journey. The car crawled through a smattering of Shropshire villages, past fields of confused cows lying in groups under the trees by the roadside. The thirty-minute journey to Shrewsbury was deathly solemn and I spent most of it gazing out the window at the thousands of plump raindrops racing down the glass, avoiding conversation.

My parents looked ahead, their eyes on the road. Occasionally, Mum would swing around to catch my eye and flash a brave smile, as much for her benefit as for mine, managing to force out a few words of reassurance to her first-born. I looked down at the swollen carrier bag of additives, colourings and sickly amounts of sugar resting between my legs. Suddenly its contents were disgusting. I slowly and methodically unwrapped a Polo mint and let it sit on my tongue, awaiting its crushing destruction. The flavour was more intense than ever.

Eventually, the emergence of glowing streetlights meant we'd hit the ring-road on the outskirts of Shrewsbury and would soon reach the hospital. What would have been a bright blue and white sign in daylight was now a smudged painter's palette of navy and reddish-purple with the Hospital's name in a bold font: Royal Shrewsbury Hospital NHS Trust. We swung a hard right into the hospital grounds. It was around 9 pm and the car park was dimly lit and quiet. The stillness was unnerving. The building spoke of the hundreds of lives that had come to an end inside its walls. Painful echoes of loved ones now departed merged with the glowing miracles of new birth and profound healing.

Walking towards the front doors, my eyes flickered left and right, seeking a swift escape. I was being led to a room where I hoped they would feed me and nurse me to the best of their abilities, provide me with laughter, drugs, and the odd bowl of apple pie and custard. The doctors would be intelligent and perky, thinking on their feet, designing me a personalised action plan.

The hospital was brightly lit and as my eyes adjusted to the shiny surfaces I took my firsts lungfuls of what I now know to be the signature 'hospital smell': distinctively sharp disinfectant alloyed with the addition of some form of inorganic perfume. Intended, I assumed, to obliterate all other odours. I'd never been to such a large hospital before.

Outside where the ambulances jerked to a halt, patients, doctors, and nurses all gathered together to smoke their cigarettes in the chilly October air. Inside it was quieter, the bustle of the day settling down into evening. My first impression was that of a glossy and depressing maze of departments, set across several different floors within multiple interconnected buildings. I felt like a trapped animal being led to the abattoir floor.

I followed my parents into the mirrored lift. A sterile cocktail of disinfectant and polish, air freshener, and sickness hung in the air. Just as the doors were threatening to clunk closed, an elfish woman in a wheelchair with sagging, jaundiced skin was wheeled in by her porter. She was mostly hairless and connected to a drip stand by a long translucent plastic wire at her wrist. Her cold eyes caught me staring at it, I blushed and quickly looked away. Soon enough that could be me.

The porter's laminated ID stated that his name was Alejo. Alejo looked full of life. He smiled and leant down to speak into her right ear.

'Come, Charlotte,' he urged with a warm Latin burr. 'We get you back to bed and I bring you nice hot chocolate, what you say?'

The woman said nothing but stared vaguely into the mid-distance, her mind seemingly part-way out of the room.

'Okay, claro, we do that then,' Alejo said, backing in and hitting six on the keypad to the right of the thick metal doors. The numeral lit up in an exotic red glow.

'Which floor for you guys?' he said, turning towards me.

'Seventh please,' said Dad. The doors sealed and clicked and the lift moved upwards. At floor six, Alejo pushed the old lady out through the doors and into a large white corridor whistling a tune none of us could place.

At the next floor, we departed the lift and walked into ward 23. Dad motioned us onward. 'They said to head straight on past ward 23 and the haematology ward is at the end.'

Immediately the smell of boiled cabbage with subtle top notes of vomit hit my nostrils. The patients here were mostly elderly and looked extremely infirm. It was hard to escape the feeling of wandering through death's waiting room. Glazed-over faces gazed from their propped-up pillows. A few nurses wandered around tending to their needs.

My heart ached, dull and heavy. How had my life come to this? It was getting towards lights-out time and the ward was winding down for the night. The patients lay gamely in bed, reading, talking to family, or just staring into space. One nurse supported an old man while he bravely hobbled to the toilet, another was sat at her desk, a clipboard face down in front of her, texting on her mobile, the edges of a smile turning up the corners of her mouth.

Towards the end of the ward was a divergent cul-de-sac containing six separate rooms. Despite its situation in the corner of a busy ward, it had a different feel, brighter, more welcoming somehow. From behind a desk, a young nurse rose to meet us. I guessed she was probably in her late twenties. Her name was Luanne and I hoped she was going to be my nurse.

'Hi, you must be Jody. Nice to meet you.'

She shook hands with my parents and flashed them a quiet, understanding smile. Behind her, a pristine whiteboard displayed the current occupants of each room like some sort of hotel, which in a way, it was. My name was written at the top of the list, on the line for room one.

'We've got your room all set up,' Luanne said. 'Follow me.'

I put my bags down on the bed and began to take in my new surroundings, scoping out the facilities in the same way you do in a holiday cottage. There was a chunky single bed on some sort of electronic piston system. Above it a grey panel, covered with switches, bulbs, pipes, and other technical-looking apparatus. Next to the bed was a side table and a jug of water. A television set nestled up in the corner on a wall mount. A small fridge and a reclinable armchair for visitors completed the picture.

My bathroom was almost as large as the room itself with a walk-in shower and finished with the classic blandness of hospital-chic decor. The moderately-sized window commanded a view over the flat rooftops of the buildings below and across to the car park. If I stood on tiptoes I could just about see the soft amber streetlights of a housing estate faintly emerging beyond the hospital gates. The realm of the free, just a few hundred metres up the driveway but a whole world away now. I had entered a bubble which required the loss of my free will. I had surrendered myself to this place and these people and their knowledge.

'Well, this is nice isn't it?' proffered Dad with a half-smile.

'Yeah, it's nicer than I was expecting,' I said. 'Does the TV have the Sky channels?'

Luanne laughed. 'No, I'm afraid our budget doesn't stretch to that, this isn't BUPA you know.'

Dad laughed. 'I'm sure he'll cope.' Everyone exchanged grateful smiles.

'Your consultant is Dr. Nigel O'Connor, he'll be along in a few minutes. He wants to do a brief check-up and talk to you about the treatment plan. You can ask him any questions, I'm sure you have plenty. I'm going to be off at eleven but Emma is the other nurse on duty, she's around somewhere and she'll be here through the night. Is there anything I can get you? A cup of tea, a glass of water maybe?'

'Oh, I'd love a cup of tea,' Dad said, motioning to Mum for her response.

'Yes thanks, that would be great.'

'Well, I'll leave you to get settled in.' Luanne let herself out, closing the door gently behind her.

Mum wandered around to inspect the bathroom and Dad helped me unpack my creased clothes and load them neatly into the tiny chest of drawers that sat next to the fridge. There was room for a medium-sized easy chair next to the bed and a normal hard-backed chair in one corner.

Luanne returned with the drinks. As she set them down on the side table there came a loud knock at the door. Without waiting for permission to enter, in swept a tall, balding gentleman in his early fifties. He was casually dressed in khaki cords and a checked shirt with his white doctor's overcoat open and flowing over the top. His squinty eyes were magnified by modest designer glasses, revealing the dull bags of one who has been working at full pelt on the absolute minimum of sleep for decades. Despite this, he was as brisk and jovial as an Army major, shaking hands with my parents, pumping their arms vigorously up and down.

'Hello. You must be Jody. How are you feeling?' he asked.

'I'm alright I guess. I'm still a bit shocked to be honest. It's all a bit overwhelming.'

'You found out today, is that right?'

'Yes, this afternoon.'

'It must have been very difficult… we're going to get you started on some chemotherapy early next week. It's best to get things rolling as soon as we can, given the severity of your condition. I'm going to take some blood from you now and check you over. Could you lie down on the bed for me – that's great– Luanne, could you fetch the trolley in for me? Thanks.

'As I'm sure you know, your white cell count is over three-hundred. This means there's something wrong with the way your blood is producing its cells. It's basically in overdrive, which is caused by cancerous cells inside you. We know it's leukaemia, which is a cancer of the blood, but it could be one of a few different types. We'll be doing some lumbar punctures to find out exactly which but from you're age and counts I'd take a guess that it's AML or ALL. They're the most common.'

'What's a lumbar puncture?'

'It's where we get a great big needle and take a sample of your bone marrow from a spot on the back of your hips.'

My face dropped at the thought of said giant needle puncturing my bones. Such dry humour. I wondered if this was the way all doctors spoke to their cancer patients? His abruptness was unnerving but it definitely broke the ice, and I could tell this gentleman was a seasoned pro in the ice-breaking business.

The doctor exchanged glances with my parents.

'Have you got any other problems?' he asked.

'I'm a bit deaf in my right ear, it's been like that for six weeks or so now. It's really annoying. I've had a cold for a while too. I keep getting large rashes all over my body. They go down in one place and then come back again somewhere else.'

'Right. Are they itchy? Raised?'

'Yeah. A little itchy and a bit lumpy, but not massively.'

'And your appetite?'

'Not too bad.'

'He hasn't been eating as much as normal,' Mum interjected.

'Ok, could you just pull your top up so I can have a feel around here. That's great, thanks.'

Snapping on a pair of beige latex gloves, he began kneading and digging into the soft flesh of my abdomen, as if searching for buried treasure. He squeezed to the left and prodded and tapped, making verbal notes to Luanne who stood beside him recording his asides. I grimaced and yelped as he hit yet another vital feeling organ.

'Spleen is enlarged. Stomach seems okay,' he continued. 'Does this hurt?' he asked, moving to the left side below my ribcage and pressing in deeply. His fingernails were just that bit too long and pinched my skin. I breathed in sharply and began what would become a continual re-evaluation of my pain threshold.

'A little,' I lied.

'Okay,' the doctor said as he removed his gloved hands from my belly.

'Luanne, would you take Jody's bloods for me please, I need to go round the other patients before I leave.

'Keep your head up Jody, we're going to help you get better. I'm not going to lie, it's going to be an incredibly tough road ahead for you. But you're a healthy young man and that instantly increases your chances of recovery. You're in the best place, we have some very good people here. I'll come by again in the morning and we can talk further; I don't want to overload you now, you've had a long day so do try and get some rest.

'Are you both staying tonight?' he asked, turning to my parents.

'I'm going to stay.' Mum said, 'Steve is going back to look after the other kids, we've got another three at home.'

'Okay, right. Good stuff. I'll leave you be. Goodnight all.'

With that Dr. O'Connor swept out of the room as swiftly as he had entered.

'He's a bit of a character isn't he?' Dad smiled.

'He is, but he's an extremely good doctor,' said Luanne. 'He's highly regarded internationally too. I've been here three years now and I can tell you that you're in very good hands.'

I felt myself tense up as waves of fearful resistance gurgled in my chest. These people wanted to invade my body. Yet clearly if I were to have any chance of survival, I would have to entrust myself to them, let them do their jobs. I didn't feel comfortable with that. It felt like giving away my power, relinquishing any remaining control over the direction of my life.

The loss of tightly held control is a wonderful leveller. Most of us grip the safety harness of our lives way too tightly. I quickly realised that my best chance of survival depended in part on my willingness to simply let go. To let go of living, to let go of dying, and surrender to any potential outcome. I would have to implicitly entrust myself to the process. I'd have to be willing to accept whatever life had in store for me through this surreal situation I was now embroiled in.

This was far from an easy task and yet I knew in my heart it was essential. I was being forced to grow up fast. I saw my parents were scared and concerned. But I also saw in their eyes a powerful sense of devotion, a plainly visible wellspring of love for their threatened first-born. Seeing this and feeling their support gave me strength. The sort of strength that allowed something a little like bravery, courage even, to emerge. It was coming from a place that felt simultaneously deep within me and yet extremely far outside of me. As such, it generated a bizarre sense of grounded detachment, as if I were treading water, my senses heightened, paradoxically aware that the outcome of this scenario depended on those around me, but to a large degree, lay in my own hands.

Late that night Dad drove home while Mum stayed with me, sleeping over in the large green armchair next to my bed, covered in a standard-issue faux-wool blanket. I'd not slept in the same room as my mother since I was a baby.

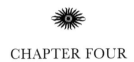

CHAPTER FOUR

Red Sky At Night

We were woken early by one of the nurses. It was around half-past seven and they were starting to serve breakfast. Hardly my normal Saturday morning routine.

'Are you decent?' came the high-pitched voice, accompanied by a sharp rapping at the door. I was lying in bed dozing. Mum was awake and reading her book. I doubt she'd got much sleep.

'Yes, we are!' she answered quickly.

A grey patent leather sandal poked its way into the room, eased the door open, and promptly propped it up with a small rubber doorstop. I could see a trolley stacked full with food trays parked outside. A short older lady was bending down to pick one out. She carried in a bowl of lukewarm oat-sludge, presented on a compartmentalised breakfast tray. Surprisingly, it didn't taste as bad as I had expected. A carton of orange juice and an underripe banana lay unopened beside it, inviting me to feed my body at least some form of nutrition.

Mary was in her early sixties, a kind-eyed Irish woman with lightly greying hair and a wit as sharp as the needles she wielded. She suffered from Addison's disease, a hormonal disorder affecting the adrenal glands and their ability to produce key hormones such as cortisol. Consequently, she only worked three shifts a week.

An extra breakfast tray for Mum was brought in, along with endless cups of tea and Mary's homemade shortbread biscuits. The lightness of her smile helped freshen the cloying atmosphere of room one. We both thought she was lovely. Mary sat on the end of my bed and happily chatted away, fielding questions about her own life and enquiring about ours. We were told how nice everyone was here. Apparently her husband had recovered from Lymphoma himself less than a year ago.

There we were, sitting in a small and very sterile room trying to maintain a vague sense of normalcy, Mum in the spongy over-sized armchair and me on the bed, eating our hospital food and taking in the saccharine monotony of breakfast TV. All sorts of tests and treatments awaited me, months of drips and drugs, and a range of unknown and potentially dangerous therapies. It felt so overwhelmingly strange, as if we'd teleported here, jumping from one life to another, and were still stunned by the whole thing, not quite believing it to be real but trying to adapt as best we could. Despite this, I felt safe and cared for, pleased that my life was in the best possible hands.

Since we'd arrived the staff had gone out of their way to make us feel at ease. The nurses we'd met were down-to-earth and genuine.

A haematology nurse must complete specialist training in order to work with patients like me and I could tell they really knew what they were talking about. I had question after question about the daily routine and the upcoming tests and procedures which they answered as best they could with care and attention. So began the slow process of learning their language.

The words buzzed around my ears like a rowdy gang of midges. Words like *lymphoblastic, chemotherapy, SATs, platelets,* and *venflon* tripped off their tongues. I wanted to know exactly what was going on; what was being done and why. This was still *my* body, with *my* cancerous blood cells inside it. Despite being slapped around the face by the stark truth of my own mortality and the fragile nature of this bag of bones that I inhabited, I still needed to exercise some sense of ownership over it. It was a small way to regain a sense of balance as the hurricane of my illness swept me up, up and away.

In the bedside drawer, my little blue Nokia 3210 vibrated with a low hum. I put down my glass of orange juice and picked it up.

From: Tash
Sent: 8:03 am
Hey you, hope you're okay. Keep smiling and I'll see you tonight. All my love xxx

It meant the world. I briefly forgot my predicament and re-read the message a few times. 'All my love.' My heart suddenly began beating a little more boldly, my cheeks flushed. I couldn't wait to see her, to hold her, and to hear her tell me everything would be alright.

The medical treatment for acute leukaemia at that time was

primarily to give several rounds of strong chemo with a potential week of radiotherapy thrown in later. Antiviral, antiemetic, and antibiotic drugs would all be given alongside at various times. Blood tests, a bone marrow sample, and several intensive scans were scheduled to happen on Monday.

A long and bumpy road lay ahead of me. Consciously or not, I had trust and faith in the system and I willingly placed myself into the care of the people whose job it was to find the best way of treating my condition. The drugs and procedures involved could be extremely debilitating to the human body and their mark might still be felt years later via a multitude of potential side effects, the most common of which is infertility. This frightened me but I knew I didn't have time to be concerned about the future. It was all happening so fast it was an effort to just stay with it and keep going.

The rest of the day passed without further consequence. The popular daytime TV show *Countdown* and a small book of crossword puzzles helped keep me sane, while the beans, boiled potatoes, and salty gammon I was given for lunch were grimly swallowed down. In the afternoon Dad returned with my younger siblings. They filed in nervously, unsure of what they'd find.

Their eldest brother was confined to a room with some weird form of cancer and they didn't know if he would even make it home again. Hugs were exchanged, eyes watered up, and another bag of supplies was emptied, milk for the fridge, juice, and snacks, the obligatory bag of grapes, and a couple of magazines. My parents, my younger sisters Jemma and Jessie, and my little brother Josh sat around my bed. It was hard for them to look me in the eye.

The family unit had been sucker-punched and was now reeling, trying to get a grip. Strangely, I felt like the strongest person in the room, just happy to be getting on with the treatment and not wishing to dwell too long in the emotional marshland of it all. They stayed until early evening and we talked about nothing and everything, but by this time Josh was getting tired so they decided to make a move. This time they were all heading home. My parents needed some time to get themselves together away from the hospital. They knew I would have to face the reality of my situation and come to terms with it by myself if I was going to have a chance of making it through. They realised I needed some space to think and to work out how I felt, to begin the mammoth task of processing the events of the last twenty-four hours.

This state of familial confusion wasn't entirely new to us, however. Three years earlier Dad had collapsed one evening in the dining room, falling to the floor quietly clutching at his chest. Mum shrieked and us kids were all scared shitless. He'd been rushed to hospital with Mum riding in the back of the ambulance. They'd diagnosed a heart attack. A completely out-of-the-blue event. He had no prior symptoms and there were no warning signs. Thankfully, he was otherwise in good health and made a full recovery. It had sent shockwaves through all of us.

That night I thought I'd lost him. I locked myself in my room and wrote what I now know to be a kind of automatic writing, my pen flying across the page, the emotions spilling out of my mind and fighting for space with salty, ink-smudged stains. I'd learned something of the power of raw grief.

That experience had taught us that life could throw some completely fucked-up situations your way and you never did know what was going to happen. There was no doubt it brought us much closer together as a family; our hearts had heard the call of separation and we'd flowered into a deeper kind of love, both consciously and unconsciously. We had come out the other side. Now, just a few years later, after things had returned to normal, here we were once more, saddened and confused, close to tears, not knowing how to proceed.

For Jemma, then aged fourteen and just hitting puberty, the impact was immediate. The evening Mum and I returned from the doctor's surgery, she was put in charge of the other two as both my parents hurriedly drove me to Shrewsbury Hospital. She had no choice but to step up, effectively becoming a part-time mother figure to the other two.

Naturally practical, Jem could cook dinner, run baths and schedule collecting little Joshy from playgroup. Even as a teenager, she was a walking, talking spreadsheet with an invaluable skillset. Over the course of my treatment, Jem somehow took on the many challenges of this heightened responsibility without grumbling or freaking out.

My younger sister Jessie had been quietly contemplative through-out. Like her little brother, she'd been processing the events and trying to deal with the shock as best she could. Her usually bright and breezy nature had dampened into something laced with enforced maturity.

Josh was only a kid, six years of age. His quiet acceptance and worried frown broke my heart each time my parents brought him to visit. Naturally, he didn't really understand what was going on and they only told him the basics: your brother is very ill and he needs to stay in the hospital for a while. He's getting special treatment and he needs us to be strong so we can help him get better. You know the sort of thing. He had no idea *how* serious it was, just that it was not simply a normal cold or virus where you spent a couple of days in bed and then you got better.

At six we are still fresh into the world, forming ideas of what's real, guided by family values as we learn the social norms. Josh's young mind was malleable and open, with no firm concept of death. I remember seeing him closely observe the looks on my parents' faces and the sombre atmosphere of tearful upset in the kitchen when Mum shared my diagnosis. Consequently, he learnt that this illness was a sad thing. Josh only knew that his older brother was suffering. What he didn't know was how to process all the thoughts and feelings flying around.

Years later, as I was starting to write this book, we all sat down together and I asked each of them to recall how they'd felt at the time of my diagnosis:

'The first time I saw you without hair in hospital you looked so different. I was so shocked, but then you smiled and I knew you were still Jody. After that people used to stop me in the high street, people who I didn't know, and ask me how you were. I always told them how strong, positive, and determined to beat it you were,' said Jemma.

Jessie remembered: 'I was just at a loss. Ever the drama queen, and so self-centred, I just kept wondering: why me? Why us? Jemma came and sat with Josh and I individually. She said to me, "It is going to be a hard few months. But I'm here. Whenever you feel sad, you come and talk to me." Back then, her words were so comforting. She was older than me, so it stood to reason that she would look after Josh and I. But now, I look back and I am in awe of her.'

For Josh, the time was less vivid but still marked a powerful moment: 'I remember sitting in the car, staring blankly out of the window while Dad and Jessie tried to explain to me what leukaemia and cancer was, but not really being able to take it in or fully understand. I just remember looking out the window full of hope that it would all be okay.'

My first love was fuelled by a fiery intensity, a level of overwhelm that blindsided me, my fragile young emotions wondering quite what the hell was happening as endorphins and dopamine mixed a mean cocktail in my heart. It marked the first time I began to learn how loving another human, outside of the family unit, could actually affect the way I lived, the choices I made and how I treated others. I discovered that a heart full of love is a kind and generous one. This helped me start crafting my own definition of what the word love actually meant. On the other hand, a supercharged first love can cast long shadows over all our subsequent relationships. We can't help but make comparisons.

Imagine then, this love of mine in full flow, its importance ramped up by my romantic teenage mind. The birds are sweetly singing their daily blessings and the world appears to dance along with the tapping rhythm of my footsteps. Life is good. No, life is *really* fucking good, perhaps the best it's ever been. Then without any real warning, suddenly everything changes. The lovestruck couple is catapulted into an extreme life-or-death experience which half-paralyses them with shock. Somehow, they attempt to forge a way through, relying on whatever emotional maturity they can muster.

There was a telephone in my room with a direct line both in and out. I'd managed to speak to Tasha briefly earlier that day.

'Morning Jode, how are you feeling today?' she asked. She sounded brave but concerned, her voice husky and perhaps a little hungover.

'Hi Tash, thanks for calling. It's weird. The doctor seems nice though, he's got a plan in mind so I'm just going to go with what he says. What else can I do?'

'I know, that sounds good. Listen, I'm getting dropped off at the hospital after the dinner round's finished around 6 pm. That still alright? It's ok if you don't feel up to it.'

'No, it's cool. I'd love that.'

'Ok, I'll see you soon.'

In truth I was feeling mixed emotions about her visit. I desperately wanted to feel the warmth of her embrace and inhale her scent. Yet I was also nervous, embarrassed that she should see me broken, diseased, and vulnerable. I could tell Tasha was scared of the situation more than she would admit. I only found out months later about how the news of my diagnosis had gone down: she'd hung up the phone and booked a taxi to The Crown, a popular pub in the town centre. There, her and Laura had got hammered on cheap bottles of Chardonnay, talking, crying, and drinking until they could do no more.

A sense of responsibility too was also slowly sinking in. Her family had been supportive but were obviously concerned. She told me her father had gently advised her not to get too close, that a relationship in this situation could just end up hurting both of us. He felt that she should support me as much as possible, but try to see me primarily as a friend. Of course, Tasha hit the roof at that. Living by her heart, going with the flow, feeling whatever came through; that was her style, never holding back, or being afraid to feel something real. A heated argument had ensued, voices were raised and Tash had spent the rest of the evening in her room with the stereo up loud, fuming.

In our short time together we'd developed a natural and easy connection that was proving to be an enjoyable exploration for our eager teenage bodies. Yet in the back of my mind lurked the natural fear that the seriousness of the situation would send her running for the hills. It would have devastated me but I could never have blamed her if she'd not been willing to stick around. Both my parents had warned me that I couldn't expect her to stay with me, that it was a potentially heartbreaking situation to take on as my girlfriend of barely two months. They said I shouldn't blame her if she decided to walk away from it all.

At five past six, I was sat watching yet another repeat of The Simpsons when her cold-blushed face appeared at the window, a nervous smile on her lips. My heart swelled in my chest. Her cheeks were flushed and I could tell she had been crying. It was an incredible relief to see her. We shared an emotional embrace and Tash made a point of kissing me firmly on the lips. Two young lovers, sat in a room while life and death watched over us.

Dealing with the surreal reality of our circumstance was not easy. Neither of us knew exactly how to act and what to say, feeling the weight of every word. We sat awkwardly on my bed and drank tea. I tried to sound positive while she took my hand and gently stroked it. I saw fear in her eyes and I saw compassion. Tasha didn't want me to die. We lay down on the bed and held each other so close I could feel the love in her heart pouring into me, warming my trembling skin and calming my racing heartbeat.

'I'm so happy you're here Tash. This is all a bit crazy isn't it?'

She stroked my hair and kissed my head and whispered into my ear, 'I'm going to be with you through all this, you know that don't you?'

My heart nearly exploded at her words, I squeezed her tighter towards me, inhaling her perfume. The dizzy rush of endorphins made me cry and smile simultaneously. What a twisted blessing to have begun a relationship with a girl like this. To know that she wanted to stay with me. She held kindness in her heart and I felt safe inside it. In her I found strength and trusted her entirely. There was love there for both of us, it was just shit timing, the absolute shittest.

After Tasha left I felt noticeably stronger, a little more relaxed. Her visit and her presence had made a difference inside me as if my own fires had been stoked by her love. Mum came back up from the canteen and asked how it went. I relayed what Tasha had said. Mum seemed happy but I don't think she quite believed it. I think she still expected her to run away from me somewhere down the line when it might all become too much. That wasn't explicitly communicated, but I could tell that's what she was thinking. My mother was just looking out for her eldest son, not wanting him to become emotionally dependant on someone who might up sticks and leave in the middle of what was clearly going to be an extremely delicate and stressful journey. I trusted Tasha, and even though I still had my doubts, in my heart I knew she'd never treat me that way, it simply wasn't in her nature.

We spoke by phone every other day, texting most days, and she came to visit whenever a lift was available. She'd bring me treats and gifts, things to make me smile, magazines, photos, CDs, snacks. She'd kiss me and hug me and tell me that everything would be okay and I believed her. Throughout the early stages of treatment I worried constantly that she would freak out and leave me. Who wants a boyfriend rapidly losing hair and bodyweight, literally wasting away, lying in a hospital bed, with his skin reeking from all the chemicals in his bloodstream? Who wants a boyfriend who can't give her pleasure or much to laugh about, take her out, and create memories together? Those kinds of thoughts tangled me up. I found it hard to trust her words, despite the glow they brought me. I had far too much time to lie in bed pondering various outcomes, to imagine where she was, what she was doing, and whom she was doing it with. On tougher days I would brace myself for a text message: 'I'm sorry. I can't do this anymore.'

Tasha was studying intensely, trying to get the grades to apply to university. She wasn't a natural academic but had other gifts by the bucketload – kind, caring, generous and hilarious, she had a natural flair for art and creative practices. Most importantly, she knew how to lift people up.

I knew it was hard on her. It was hardest for all of those around me. But somehow Tash never felt that being with me was too much responsibility. She was a heart-on-her-sleeve kind of girl. She'd said she'd be there for me and so, she was. A commitment had been made and her intent was clear. Though it must have been shocking and intimidating, Tash never appeared fazed by my appearance, my vomiting, or the variety of weird smells that permeated my room. Knowing that on her visits she'd more often than not snuggle up on the bed with me was nothing less than a fiery beacon of hope.

To feel her presence, both visible and invisible, brought me incredible strength and solace at the very worst of times. She helped pull me through. With her open-heart, she bolstered me and helped me to connect to the reserves of strength and focused positivity deep inside. Talking to her now, Tash tells me how my courage was an inspiration, my sense of calm amazed her, and that she deeply admired the bravery I showed. All I know is that she gave her love to a shrunken teenage boy when it absolutely mattered, and for that I am forever grateful.

CHAPTER FIVE

Lumbar Puncture

Monday. Tasha had left for a scheduled geography field trip in mid-Wales. I would have to be content with the sound of her voice for a week and hopefully a few texts. The group would return a week later, by which time I would be fully immersed in my first chemotherapy regime, most probably shitting and vomiting and shedding hair all over the place if what I'd been told was even half-true. Not the best setup for a hot date with your new girl, but it would have to do.

The first week of my new existence brought a multitude of tests and procedures to submit to. The MRI and CT scans involve you being placed inside those giant polo mint machines you sometimes see on films and TV. Strangely, it was actually quite exciting to experience such a futuristic process. I had the realisation that human ingenuity is responsible for developing these insanely complex contraptions, devices capable of producing incredibly detailed images of my internal tissues, organs, and blood vessels. Through the use of special dyes, they can actually follow the flow of blood around. To get scanned by one is also extremely daunting, linked as they inevitably are with cancer, tumours, and serious health concerns. You kind of know that something isn't quite right if you have to get in one.

The technicians get you to lie down on a human-sized baking tray which then slides smoothly inside the machine. The CT scanner uses X-ray radiation so you have to hold your breath while the machine does its thing. The MRI was to scan my brain. First, they asked me to drink a small cup of tasteless liquid, then after a short time, they used the big machine to follow the visual signature of this liquid as it traveled around inside the body. This enabled them to build up a detailed image which they then examined for further diagnostic information.

Blood tests were a daily occurrence. When I'd arrived, they'd put in a temporary needle called a cannula, commonly referred to as a venflon. This was inserted into a vein on the top of my left hand and then taped over to keep it there. This enabled them to give me fluids as well as take blood samples without having to break the skin each time. Unfortunately, my veins just were too weak to keep them in for long periods, so every other day I'd need them to put in a fresh one. Venflons by necessity have quite long needles and having them inserted was generally a pretty unpleasant experience. When one of my regular nurses – Luanne, Emma, or Mary – took charge the process was over quite quickly without too much discomfort on my part.

One afternoon when it was time for a new cannula, a junior

doctor that I'd never met before was instructed to take on the job. I became the rather unwilling guinea pig to this plainly nervous young student who couldn't have been more than a couple of years my senior. The poor guy struggled with my fading veins for over half an hour. Each time he failed, his face went a shade redder. I became more and more irritated by all the pain and his incompetence, beginning to feel like a human pin cushion. After about the fourth or fifth failed attempt I lost it, and screamed at him to get out and get someone in who could actually do the job. Hearing the commotion, Mary came rushing in and within two minutes she'd got me all fixed up. I never saw that particular junior doctor on the haematology ward again.

Thankfully, the venflons were not a long-term solution. Dr. O'Connor (henceforth to be referred to by our nickname for him – Doc Oc) had mentioned early on that I'd need to have a line put in and had explained to us what that meant. A Hickman line is a thin flexible plastic tube that is inserted under anaesthetic into one of the main arteries in your chest to help streamline the process of receiving drugs and other fluids. It was a pre-requisite for delivering my first round of chemotherapy, which was scheduled to start soon after.

He assured me it would be a simple procedure for the guys down in theatre. I'd be under anaesthetic and would barely notice, he said, in his typically nonchalant way. The doctor had a knack of referring to these sorts of things as if they were easy and trivial. His confidence inspired my own. No doubt it was a well-practised technique of his. It was easy to think, 'Well, if the doc says it's that simple, what is there to worry about?'

I prepared myself for the surgery by putting on a funny little dressing gown. It was extremely thin, and a sickly shade of washed-out turquoise. For the big event, they opened both doors to my room and wheeled me out through the ward and down a couple of levels in the lift to the theatre. I lay back on my bed, slightly bemused by the whole thing. I felt like the Queen on a royal visit. Allowed out of the hallowed walls of my palace under strict supervision and chauffeured along to my destination. Heading down to have a bunch of men in masks cut my chest open was not quite such a glamorous occasion, however, although part of me did enjoy the surreal novelty of it all and couldn't help but let out a nervous laugh.

They wheeled me straight into the operating room on my bed and locked the wheels down. I looked up into the bright lights and saw a group of three or four people leaning over me, all clad in surgical scrubs and masks. All I could see were their eyes and a few stray clumps of hair. I think one of them was a woman. They said they were going to give me a sedative and that I should begin to count to ten.

'One... Two... Threeee... Fo...'

Fade to black in a warm rush of chemicals. I was out. Swimming in a bottomless pool of darkness.

But not for long. From some murky dreamworld of shadows and metallic sound, my bleary eyes opened. It was so bright. Dark shapes moved around above me and I felt an extremely strange sensation in my chest. Lifting my head slightly, I managed to look down and catch a blurred snapshot of the scene, mid-insertion:

'Whhhaaaaat thaa fuuuck...?'

'More sedative please,' came the robotic response, the voice floating somewhere behind me.

In a few more seconds I dissolved into blackness again.

I awoke in my room to find myself sat upright, propped up on a neatly arranged three-pillow stack, the covers wrapped around my body and a flimsy, semi-translucent white gown around my skin. I must have missed the return bed-taxi journey completely. I looked down at my chest from where a dull throbbing was emanating. I peeled back one side of my gown to reveal a white plastic tube dangling from underneath a thick square of gauze, secured along each side by the sticky glue of medical tape. Intrigued at the sight of this inorganic tube connecting with the bloody pipes inside my body, I flicked its red and blue-capped ends without thinking. They swished around like a donkey's tail swatting summer flies, causing a shudder of pain to shoot down my right side.

I didn't feel like getting up but couldn't ignore the aching twinge in my bladder from the half-litre of hot urine that had been held back by my comatose state for nearly two hours. Limping slightly, my stiff muscles adjusted to their first real use of the day and carried me to and from the toilet and back onto my bed. My mouth was dry, I needed a glass of water. Minutes passed in silence.

After a short time, in which I was successfully able to doze off, the door handle turned gently downwards and Mum crept back into the room, easing it shut behind her. She sat down in the easy chair and opened the copy of *The Times* she had brought in with her, placing her latest plastic cup of tea down on the table beside the bed, being careful not to make too much noise. My sleep was only a by-product of the remnants of the anaesthetic in my system, the body resting itself to rebuild the cells around the wound that ultimately would allow me a better chance at survival.

I came round again later that afternoon. Emma said not to open the large square dressing taped to my skin, or get water on it for at least another twenty-four hours, but the next time I went to the bathroom I couldn't resist. I could feel the plastic tube inside my chest which was new and bizarre and made my toes curl. Peeling back the tape, wincing as hairs were ripped out at their tiny roots, I saw the nozzle end of the thin white line hanging limply against my chest which was bruised yellow and still stained faintly with iodine.

I looked at myself in the long mirror on the wall. Reality check. There were plastic tubes dangling out of my chest and I was soon to be dosed with one of the most toxic substances known to medicine. I had cancer in my bloodstream. I might soon die. Things had got pretty fucking weird pretty quickly. I felt like I was hallucinating. It still didn't feel real and part of me expected to simply wake up and get back to the day-to-day happenings of teenage life. I took a few deep breaths. Looking into my own worried eyes I promised myself I would fight. I couldn't allow this disease to take my future away.

With the line installed they could now start delivering all the different substances which were required as part of my treatment. In conjunction with a drip machine to control the flow, I would be given bags of blood, platelets, saline solution, a variety of high-strength antibiotics, antifungals, and antiemetics as well as my chemotherapy. Doc Oc had said from the get-go they needed to begin chemo as soon as possible to give me the best chance of staying alive. At the time I didn't give this much of a second thought. I knew I was ill,

I knew it was serious. Only many years later would Mum finally let slip that on the night I was admitted, he'd taken her and Dad aside. He'd told them gravely that my white blood cell count was so high that without any intervention I only had a couple of weeks of life left. After that my body would begin to shut down and death would be inevitable.

Taking a bone marrow sample, a *lumbar puncture* as they called it in the trade, was a key aspect of my treatment. It allowed them to see how everything was functioning inside my bones and my spinal fluid. The first time they did it, Doc Oc said they would use a local anaesthetic.

'Ahhh, there's nothing to worry about, it's not too bad,' he said. I swear I saw a mischievous glint in his eye.

I went along with that but let me tell you now, when a long thick needle that looks like something one might use to pacify a horse is wheeled out and subsequently inserted deep into the base of your spine, it is extremely fucking uncomfortable. The bizarreness of the sensation was striking. A new kind of bodily penetration was being performed upon me. It made me cry out loud with the pain, even after the anaesthetic. The base of my back was tight, bruised, and worryingly sore for a day or two afterwards. I could barely stand up straight, gaining a clear insight into the plight of the elderly, hobbling to the loo and back bent over like a wizened old man. After that, I vowed to take Doc Oc's breezy nonchalance with a pinch of salt and to always ask for the full knockout dose of midazolam whenever I wanted it.

I grew to rather like the midazolam. With life in the balance, I took my fun where I could get it. I am in no way suggesting that this drug is a recreational experience. It is very much not. It can put you on your back in less than ten seconds. I know this as I was always instructed to count backwards from ten and never once made it past five. It pulled my consciousness away into a sweetly medicated sleep, from which I would awaken feeling giddy and silly, not yet attuned to the pain emanating from my lower back. It was through these experiences that I came to understand how people can get addicted to opiates. When life is painful, the sugary sweet totality of absolute numbness can feel like ecstasy.

The results of all my various scans and tests came back as rapidly as you might expect when a young life hangs in the balance. Chemotherapy was planned for the next day. They actually started the treatment before really knowing exactly what sort of leukaemia I had. Things were that serious.

My treatment plan consisted of two week-long treatments followed by another week's recovery time. I'd get a week in my room to let my body adjust and recover while taking IV bags of antibiotics and antiemetics, and necking down the handfuls of vitamin and mineral tablets they brought round every morning. This was to allow my healthy white cells a chance to re-grow and some small level of immunity to return once I was out of the dangerous neutropenic stage.

Being neutropenic means the blood is devoid of neutrophils, a type of white blood cell that forms the first line of defence for the immune system. If all went to plan, I'd even be allowed to go home for five days or so at the end of each cycle but it was far from guaranteed. There would be a strict list of restrictions attached to any home visits that I would have to adhere to.

From: Tash
Sent: 9:14 pm
Hope it went ok today Jode. Thinking of you.
Love T xxx

It was mid-October and the days hadn't yet turned frosty. The sun continued to shine, bringing much-needed illumination to my dark and cancerous corner of the world. Just another teenage boy ensconced in his room. I wondered how many others like me there were around the world. In the exact same situation, at the exact same time, somehow bound together by misfiring and confused bone marrow. Across the hospital car park, the trees proudly displayed a hundred shades of rusted copper. Their autumn leaves drifted to the ground, gracefully accepting an unavoidable death.

Besides Doc Oc, the first people I had come into contact with on ward 23 were the specialist haematology nurses. They manned a small reception area in front of the six private rooms, working in small rotating teams of two or three, depending on how many patients were in the rooms. Each and every one of the nursing team who cared for me on that ward were very special human beings, but Emma and Luanne quickly became my favourites.

For a testosterone-fueled teenager at the brink of manhood, Luanne, with her cropped hair and smiling blue eyes, sparked a 'hot blonde nurse' fantasy. In this sterile environment, her bubbly nature was nothing short of a gift. That she was sweet and caring with a heart of gold just made it all the more perfect. Dad grew pretty fond of her too, practising his ridiculous flirting technique at every opportunity, which was often as hilarious as it was embarrassing.

Emma, who must have been around the same age, was the cool big sister I never had. We shared a similar sense of humour and a love of music. She was quirky, laid back, and an asset to the team. I fondly remember many quiet night shifts where she'd come and sit at the foot of my bed. All the other patients were asleep so she'd pop into my room for a chat.

'You buzzed me, Jody,?' she said, poking her head around the door.

'Sorry Emma, would you be able to get me a jug of iced water please? My mouth is so sore again.'

'Of course, be right back.' She disappeared, returning a few minutes later with a big jug and a glass, setting them down on my side table. I took a big gulp, holding the chilled water in my mouth for a few seconds before swallowing.

'How are you doing?' she asked.

'I ache all over and the inside of my cheeks are blistered. It's pretty shit,' I replied honestly.

'Chemo is notorious for mouth ulcers. If the pain gets too much let me know and I'll get you something to help you sleep.'

'Ah, thanks Emma.'

'That's what I'm here for. So anyway, I hear you're a drummer?'

'Yeah that's right. Or perhaps I used to be.' I grimaced.

'And you shall be again!' she declared, grinning. 'What do you want to do when all this over? When you can go out in the world again?'

'Well, I've never been to a music festival, that'd be amazing. I keep hearing Glastonbury is fun. And, I'd like to get a tattoo I think.'

'A tattoo? Cool, well you'll have to wait until you're properly better for that but festivals are brilliant. Me and Ian go to Glastonbury every year and we have a right old time.' She shot me an exaggerated wink.

In those moments it felt like I had real friends with me, they kept me positive and lifted my thoughts without promising anything or trying to be a counsellor. The only difference being that these real-life angels were there for me 24/7. Such devotion to caring. They knew plenty about my condition and the treatments I would be facing. My parents and I must have asked them so many repetitive questions but every time they politely and patiently went into detail when they answered and tried not to candy-coat the truth. I appreciated that. I trusted them. I have so much to thank them for.

Mary was the elder of the crew, she did fewer shifts than the others and as such wasn't around as often, but we all enjoyed her presence, my parents especially. She had a wicked sense of humour, extremely dry but without any trace of nastiness. Her heart was always right there on her sleeve and that was why we liked her. There wasn't much that was off-limits. She kept me laughing and on my toes, pulling me out of sinking introspection with her biting wit and no-bullshit attitude.

From the moment I was diagnosed, normal family life was flattened into the earth. The strength and courage that emerged from amidst the fear and confusion of our family unit was humbling. You never know how strong you are until you are truly put to the test. Forced to face an almost insurmountable challenge with your back firmly against the wall. I knew there was a deep bond of love between us. I'd been on the receiving end of it since I was a kid.

The way our family faced my illness was a clear demonstration of how love can be seen as the willingness to sacrifice personal needs for those of another, especially when the shit really hits the fan. It taught me that love is the ability to understand where the collective priorities are, and to respond accordingly when they shift and change. Love is also accepting the care and support of others, allowing yourself to be loved. Allowing yourself to be rocked, held, and spoken to softly when all around you, life appears to be in the process of a great demolition and dusty clouds obscure your future. As humans, our potential for commitment to each other in moments of deep stress and trembling fear can be nothing short of magical, whether blood relatives or absolute strangers.

By now, most of my year-group were aware of the illness I was fighting. My parents had phoned to make the head teacher aware and an announcement had been made. I'd told my friends Rob and Ben just after it happened and they called or text me every week to see how I was, relaying the updates back to everyone at school. None of them had been to see me yet; I wasn't ready to face anyone outside of Tasha and my family. At my request, she'd given a short progress update to the common room, letting everyone know how I was doing and how they might show their support by writing me a card or buying me a few small items.

You could say I was a minor school celebrity, albeit an invisible one, sheltered from the limelight by mystery. Tash told me that people would come up to her almost daily. Concerned classmates and teachers stopped her in the corridors, or outside of school hours when she was walking through the town. They all wanted to know how I was doing, if I was ok. People cared. The grim spectre of disease had touched everyone's lives by its presence in one of their own.

Life as I knew it, with all its colourful details and routines, had begun to retreat. My world was shrinking. For now, it encompassed only these hospital walls. Visitors were transported to my little island of flashing LEDs and steadily bleeping drip machines, complete with the familiar whiff of bleach and lingering lunchtime curry.

I can state with complete sincerity the profound gratitude I have for being birthed into the very family that I needed around me when all this insanity came whirling onto the doorstep of our cosy home. My three brave siblings and two indomitable parents showed me their hearts and gave up a hell of a lot for me.

Their coping mode was highly efficient. Years spent juggling full-time teaching careers, four young kids and a dog, had somewhat prepared them for emergencies; quickly shifting gears to help us navigate through tough times.

As I became the priority, Mum and Dad spent most of their time either working, visiting me, or attempting to continue with normal family life. They'd initially been signed off for a month each, with Mum given assurances that she could take all the time she needed after that. Adding to the stress, Dad faced some tough negotiation with his Headteacher to receive the same level of support. This now meant that they could alternate their daily visits without tiring themselves out. That in itself was incredible.

Knowing they were there for me whenever I needed them was reassuring and gave me something solid to hold onto, even if they were barely holding it together. The illusion of unbreakable strength would certainly have shattered had I been able to see beyond my own perspective.

My parents' loving presence provided a container, a cocoon of safety and support, within which I could open into the experience. They helped me understand what was happening and eased my transition into my new surroundings. They listened when I needed to talk and never pressured me when I couldn't find the words. Even if I'd died within the first couple of weeks of diagnosis, my soul slipping away to some other place, I knew in my heart that I was truly held by them. I felt the raw honesty of their love. Isn't that really all that anyone can hope for when death is close: to be held and loved unconditionally?

Mum and Dad had to press pause on their own lives, and to a degree even those of the other kids. Looking back, they wish they could have done certain things differently. But what choice did they have? All I know is, my family did their damn best and I love them for it.

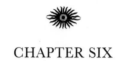

CHAPTER SIX

Operation Cell Death

The process of chemotherapy treatment began with me lying back on my bed. First, my Hickman line was flushed with saline solution by one of the nurses, a standard procedure. Meanwhile, someone proudly wheeled in a trolley carrying a large transparent bag of Mediterranean-blue liquid. Hung from a metal stand, its contents would steadily drip into my body over the next few hours.

The bag was housed in a thick plastic casing, and sported an icon of a black cross on an orange background, which indicated that this was some serious shit. I tried not to think about all the side-effects and the damage that it could cause, and instead worked to view it as a healing liquid. If this procedure had any chance of working I felt I must be willing to reframe my experience. Simultaneously poison and medicine, these luminous bags would grow to become my allies. From my hospital bed I learnt the bitter joy of paradox.

After Doc Oc finished briefing me, he flipped the switch on my drip stand to let the first bag of mitoxantrone into my bloodstream. Its mission was to wipe out as many dividing blood cells as it could – a killing machine in liquid form. Strangely, it was comforting, reminding me of the Blue Cola *Panda Pops* I'd buy from the corner shop on my way home from school.

Mum and Dad sat with me as the drip…drip…drip…drip of azure liquid made its way inside me, spreading out into my bloodstream and pumping around my body like a nuclear daiquiri, all guns blazing, as Operation Cell Death formally commenced.

I'd been listening to Britrock band Feeder a lot since being admitted, as they'd recently released their second album, *Yesterday Went Too Soon*. In the days before the vast catalogues of smartphone streaming and MP3 players, I only had a few CDs and consequently, it had gained pretty heavy rotation on my shitty little stereo. I tested Mary's patience with the volume. Occasionally she'd stick her head around the door, fix me with her best stern-not-stern look and ask me politely but firmly to turn it down. Some things never change. The opening track, 'Anaesthetic', with its simple, chiming refrain always made me think of Tasha and the effect she was having on my attitude to the whole experience.

The punchy indie-rock that album delivered was an oddly fitting soundtrack to the tumult in my inner world during that time. It was as if it had been written just for me, a sequence of simple songs to help get me through each day.

Whether it was Richard and Judy fooling around with meaningless content on *This Morning*, or Dad's favourite celebrity mathematician Carol Vorderman on *Countdown*, the TV provided a welcome distraction. The fourteen-inch screen offered a window into the world outside my room. The banality of daytime programming took us away from the critical procedure going on right beside my bed. It gave me and my parents a break from having to think or talk about everything that was happening. Instead, we could just laugh along at the antics, take a sip of tea and for a few seconds, briefly forget.

After twenty-four hours I didn't feel too bad, a little tired perhaps. The nauseous ache around my stomach was disconcerting but not yet uncomfortable. A second and third day of treatment passed and I began to feel properly woozy. My appetite started to noticeably decrease. That week continued in much a similar rhythm. Steadily-dripping bags did their murderous work. I continued to seek relief in the constant hum of daytime television.

On one of my bathroom missions, I took a pre-shower piss only to see a stream of alarmingly dark blue urine. My armpits smelt rancid yet also a little sweet, no doubt the result of my liver and kidneys working away to process the stack of drugs and keep the rest of my body functioning.

At the end of five full days of intensive chemotherapy, my appetite disappeared entirely. The nurses coaxed me to chug down sludgy, nutrient-dense liquid meals twice a day, the consumption of which I can only liken to a mildly fruity, finely-powdered carpet cleaner, mixed with the pulp of some on-the-turn blackcurrants and diluted with heavily-chlorinated tap water. As if to spite me further, I was having trouble holding the bastards down. These regular toilet dashes flushed away what little energy I had left.

I have had trouble swallowing pills and tablets since I was young. My throat would tighten, the tablets would get stuck and I'd freak out, semi-choking. It was a self-fulfilling prophecy which I've now thankfully, for the most part, overcome.

After several near-misses with ludicrously gigantic capsules and pressed pills, the nurses delivered a special little pill-crushing device, designed for those truly unable to swallow. This small circular grinder ground the pills into dusty fragments that I would then mix into water or sprinkle on my food like some sort of high-grade medicinal condiment. This worked for a short while but quickly became more hassle than it was worth as my appetite further decreased. The nausea, combined with not feeling hungry and the distinctly average nature of the hospital food, meant another way would have to be found. When a plate of bland, overcooked baked beans, topped with powdered potassium (the bitterest, most effective taste-destroyer) is placed in front of you, it's a certain kind of torture.

Eventually, after a couple of pained requests, a kind employee at the pharmacy took pity on me and created special liquid versions of these pills. This wasn't something that already existed, so they had to make each one from scratch especially for me – the absolute saints. I was so relieved, grateful not to have to force down cold, potassium-laced baked beans ever again.

Over the slow days that followed, I grew progressively thinner, weaker, and much sicker. The vomiting began in earnest one Thursday afternoon while I sat watching another *Perry Mason* repeat. During a challenging lunch consisting of half a vile carpet-shake and two brave mouthfuls of beans on toast, I felt the urgent jolt of my stomach wanting to simply get rid...get rid...GET RID. Powerless to stop myself, the contents sprayed across the bed, my food tray, and the floor. It felt like a layer of skin peeled off, as a torrent of purple and red goo formed a viscous pool, slowly inching its way towards the door. It left my throat stinging with the whip of the sharpest bile. I slammed the black button above my bed with the vague icon of a nurse printed on it. This triggered a red light on a board next to the nurses' desk telling whoever was on duty which room's occupant was in need of urgent assistance.

At this point, I was expelling at least two lots of vomit a day. Weakness had descended to the very core of my bones as the drugs worked their way deep into my system. My muscles began to melt away and my skin hung from my shoulders like a pallid cape. I had severe cramp along my shins, and raw sores had erupted along the fleshy insides of my cheeks. On one occasion, while watching Carol sashay around with her big plastic letters, Dad encouraged me to try a small amount of fruit. A sole white grape triggered a mouthful of watery stomach contents. Mum stroked my back with a grimace as I ruined my bedsheets yet again and wondered what the fuck was happening inside my body.

The nurses tried to combat the severe sickness with antiemetic drugs but the multitude of tablets had begun to turn my fragile stomach into a reactive pit of chemical soup. I resolved to nibbling on chunks of ginger root, relieving the nausea a little. It was debilitating but the one positive I could see was that the chemo seemed to have fixed my partial deafness. One day, when talking with Tasha on the phone about the gossip from her field trip, I was suddenly delighted to find that my hearing was back to normal. Sound was open and full again. Voices were not muffled and I was no longer straining myself to hear. It was an ironic and short-lived happiness.

My view was very much 'just get in there and do your work, drugs' and so that was how the second week continued. Another day, another bag. Another TV show, another spin of my Feeder CD. Take a breath and let it in.

It was a tense few days waiting for the neutrophil count to rise. They can make up to 70% of the white blood cells that form our body's first line of defence against any invading bacteria and parasites. First on the scene, they are extremely important in the way our bodies deal with any incoming challenges or threats. Once these cells had recovered to levels above the required threshold, the nurses promised I could be allowed out of my room. It was also possible that they wouldn't. If that happened I'd be stuck there in the same room until the next round started.

Thankfully my neutrophil count slowly crept up. The freedom to roam was almost mine. Initially, my territory was limited to ward 23. At the very end, there was a small stark sitting room, comprised of a TV and two almost comfortable sofas. Despite this, being there felt utterly momentous.

For my first outing, Mum wheeled me down to the hospital cafe for a weak cup of tea. As excited as I was to finally leave my little magnolia box, containment had left me with a deep empathy for any being who spends the majority of their day confined within four walls. It's no kind of life.

One afternoon, a few of my school mates came to visit. They brought me snacks, books, and a couple of films to watch. Their joking and laughing grounded me and took me out of my head. I enjoyed them filling me in on the latest gossip from school, but as we spoke I felt myself drifting away from that life. After they left, I realised I might never hang out with them like we used to again. Their lives would continue on a different trajectory, while mine was dramatically on hold. I'd always be different to them, forever changed.

My astronomical, life-threatening white-cell count had been tamed by the first round of chemo. My neutrophil count had risen enough for them to be happy for me to spend a weekend at home and so Mum collected me and we drove back to Bridgnorth.

I remember hobbling to the car in the hospital car park and thinking that at any moment a nurse would come sprinting out of the front doors to call me back inside. I hadn't been there since the day of my diagnosis and so much had happened in that time. Around three weeks had passed since I was admitted but it felt like months.

A Hickman line hung limply from my chest. I'd lost several kilos in weight. The vomiting and diarrhoea had calmed a little but my diet was severally restricted and I could still feel the remnants of poison running around in my veins. They gave me a drip stand and a few bags of saline to take home, as well as a white paper bag stuffed full of different coloured pills. I was given strict instructions to flush my line regularly to stop any blood clotting and to keep the dressings clean.

Walking into the house, I immediately shed a layer of fear. Mac ran up to me, wagging his bushy white tail like a dog possessed. He jumped up, pressing his soft pads onto my thighs, his eyes dancing with happiness, and excitedly covered my bare arms with wet dog licks. Mum scolded him. We used to rough and tumble, but now even this show of affection could easily have knocked me over. Regaining my balance, I laughed and dug my fingers deep into his pure white coat, ruffling him up and scratching him behind his ears, treasuring that famous dopey grin.

Welcomed back into the bosom of the family nucleus with smiles and hugs aplenty, I lay upon the settee, sipping a herbal tea. My inquisitive siblings sat around, asking all kinds of questions about my treatment and how I was feeling, whilst in the kitchen Mum clinked cutlery and chopped vegetables in a cloud of aromatic steam. A homecoming dinner was being prepared. Everything I liked best. We were to have corn on the cob to start, warm from the pot and drenched in butter, followed by a hearty shepherd's pie with steamed vegetables from Dad's garden to be liberally doused with a rich leek gravy. Proper British soul food.

I gained much solace that night from the simple pleasure of watching television with my family, all of us gathered together in the front room with the dog snoozing on the rug at our feet, and trying very hard to feel normal. The first time I was allowed to leave the hospital was bittersweet. It felt so strange to be back at home in what were extremely familiar surroundings in the wider context of a very unfamiliar set of circumstances, with my family all looking at me differently, constantly checking on me, living their lives around me.

The next day, I rested and waited for Tasha. In the late afternoon I checked my watch for the third time in ten minutes and felt a tingling glow spread out across my body. She was coming over that evening. Eventually the doorbell rang. Jessie dashed ahead to open the door and Tasha came bounding in, light shining from her eyes and a shower-fresh smell. We embraced in the hallway, Mac fussing at her feet, then quickly decamped up to my room.

The cream storage heater purred away in the corner. We lay back on my single bed, as I ran my fingers through her hair the way people do in films. Tasha looked at me, her eyes flickered slightly, wet at the edges. She moved her mouth towards mine in what felt like the first real kiss of my life. The barriers of disease and distance briefly dissolved.

We spent the next couple of hours with our limbs entwined, feeling each other's heat under the glow of the TV. We watched a film, ate handfuls of sugary popcorn, and enjoyed our first normal evening together in what felt like months. Soon after Tash left in a taxi, I fell into a deep, contented sleep.

From: Tash
Sent: 11:57 pm
So good to see you tonite Jodybear,
you're my hero! Speak soon. Love T xxx

Returning to hospital was depressing in the extreme. Back to my small room, to the poisonous drip bags and another punishing couple of weeks of chemotherapy. Back to the familiar and rotten side-effects. That short break home had been a worthy tonic. Seeing Tash briefly and spending precious time with my family had helped stabilise the darkness in my imagination, tempering my despairing thoughts.

Doc Oc came around one evening as I was settling down to watch yet another episode of *Eastenders*. I didn't even like the show, it just helped bring the largeness of the outside world into my own. Usually, the good doctor breezed into my room with some quip about my food or a band he'd heard on the radio on his way to work. Today he wasn't quipping and he definitely wasn't breezing. Entering slowly and closing the door precisely behind himself, he sat down on the edge of my bed and came right out with it.

'So Jody, good to see you. Did you enjoy your time at home?'

'Yes, it was great to eat some real, good food again,' I said.

'Is that so,' said the doctor. 'Well Jody as you know, the plan was to do three courses of dual chemotherapy, under the impression that you've got acute lymphoblastic leukaemia (ALL), which you have markers to suggest. We've received some more details back from the lab today that reveal you actually show markers for both ALL and acute myeloid leukaemia (AML). Now don't worry, this shouldn't change things too much overall, but it does mean we need to change the type of drugs we're using. One of them, in particular, is slightly stronger than you may have been used to and its side effects can be more pronounced, so I have to warn you about that.'

'What sort of symptoms? The same ones I've been having, the vomiting, mouth sores and all of that?'

'Yes, you'll find that you will lose your hair more quickly, and you may experience muscle wasting, diarrhoea and eczema. We'll be able to help you keep a lid on these things but it will be more important the next time you go home that you really avoid any contact with germs or bacteria. Your immune system will be almost down to nothing.'

'Oh. Ok.'

'It should start to recover again, don't worry, but we may need to keep you in for a week or two longer before you can leave. We've got to play it by ear and see how your body copes. Do you understand all that?'

'Yeah. I think so.'

'Well, next time your parents are in, I'll make sure to explain it to them again with you here. But don't be disheartened, you're doing really well. We think you're making excellent progress. We'll just need to monitor your cell activity closely to see how the treatment is working, and I know you don't like them but we also need to take another lumbar puncture next week to analyse your spinal fluid. You can swear if you like.'

'Fuck!' I knew what was in store.

'Exactly,' he laughed, 'but like last time I will be doing it myself and you'll be under sedation, so no need to worry.'

'Ok. Well, I guess I've got no choice but to keep on keeping on,' I replied, yet again submitting myself to whatever they needed.

'That's the spirit,' Doc Oc said, patting his thigh earnestly as he rose. 'I'll drop by again tomorrow, if you think of anything you want to ask me I shall do my best to answer. I'll leave you to your *Eastenders*.'

'Actually, I hate it.'

'Yes, it's awful isn't it. I suggest you watch something better! See you later.' The doctor slipped from the room and I was alone once again.

Part Two

INITIATION

*Having traversed the threshold, the hero moves in
a dream landscape of curiously fluid, ambiguous
forms, where he must survive a succession of trials*

Joseph Campbell

Ω

The Cowboy

With his battered hat pulled low, the wide rolling brim concealed his face – a sweep of greying stubble across tanned and ageing skin the only visible feature. It was dawn and the sun was not yet up. Too risky to travel without it, so he parked Dusty, his 1973 Winnebago Brave, under a small grove of Sweet Acacia trees. He dropped the passenger seat back, settling in to it's creased leather, softened by regular siestas. Outside the window, waving cacti and blurred horizon lines hummed a sweet desert lullaby.

Dusty was a proud and reliable machine. Desert driving had been his baptism, his graduation, and the source of his decay, but stick your head through the side door and you'd see his best days were not yet behind him. The panoramic windscreen flaunted vibrant orange curtains, tied back neatly on either side. A matching burnt orange shag carpet lined the cabin floor. He carried the magnificent honour of a retired knight returning to battle. Though his once-sparkling chrome was now dull and forgiving, flecked with dings and scratches, plenty of life waited in the pipes and bolts of his eager engine.

As Dusty kept watch, his partner dozed. The lilac clouds high above the scrub drifted with the steady rhythm of his breathing. Further out, beyond the dramatic peaks that formed the North-Western boundary, the sky was bruising indigo. A towering outcrop of volcanic memory stood proud among pine forested slopes. Shadows slid between the tree trunks, avoiding the rising light. In the ancient riverbed below, the sound of scuttling scorpions encouraged the rains to fall. A gang of wasps the size of a fist dodged in and out of a bleached-dry trunk, while three black crows screeched a war cry, eyeballs dangling from sockets, their feathers clumped together with an oily slickness.

After a short time, the old man stretched out slowly like a cat and sat up. He slapped his face with practised rigour and drew back the curtains. Way off in the distance the storm clouds gathered above the peaks. They seemed angry, bloated with the desire to let loose all that they carried.

'Fuck... ah well, he'll be here soon. Time to hit the road Dusty.' He struck the dashboard as if cajoling a grumpy mule. Dusty gurgled from a whisper to a roar in response.

I took a lift from the hospital lobby to the fourth floor and wandered slowly back to my room, the fuzzy glow of happiness engulfing me.

Life felt fluid. I stretched myself out on the familiar dumpy bed – a short nap was called for.

An attractive blonde nurse in a revealing uniform came by to check my blood pressure. As she bent over to pick up a cuff from her trolley, I saw there was nothing beneath her white dress. A dopey grin swamped my teenage face; this was just too good to be true... and it really fucking was.

She flew at me, teeth bared, snarling like a rabid dog. In her hand was a needle as long as my forearm. She held it like a dagger, stabbing down frantically, aiming for my flesh but missing as I kicked my legs out of the way. Catching her full in the face with a sweeping right foot, I knocked her back onto the floor, dazed. Time enough for me to hop off the bed and get the hell out of there.

Low down on the wall behind my bed, amid all the sockets and wires, a small door swung open invitingly. It barely seemed large enough for me to crawl through, but the image of that great needle coming at my rear end generated more than enough adrenalin to get me shifting. Pyjama-clad and heart racing, I went for it, slamming the door shut behind me.

Breathing heavily, eyes adjusting to the blinding light, I found myself on the summit of a small sand dune. I rose to my feet and dusted myself off, spitting out the few grains that had inevitably found their way into my mouth. I looked around. The small door had vanished. Nothing but desert in every direction. A vast expanse under a limitless sky. The sun hung high, telling me that the day in this place was far from over. The land below was dotted with brown-green bushels and crisscrossed by a few solitary vehicle tracks. On the horizon, I could just about make out the blueing tips of a mountain range above which the clouds were gathering in. They looked like the spine of a sleeping dragon. A wooly sense of amnesia taunted me, daring me to figure out exactly why I was stood in the middle of a landlocked sea of sand, in my pyjamas, with no logical explanation for how I'd arrived.

'Ahoy there!'

I wouldn't say the voice was near enough to be described as loud, but a few feet closer and it would have been yelling in my ear. I spun around to see a classic American Winnebago, painted deep Lapis Lazuli blue, idling at the side of a dust-streaked road that skirted the dunes, before veering off towards the mountains. Neither the van, nor the road, were there a few seconds earlier, yet both were right in front of me now, real as life. The van's meaty engine turned over with the hunger of a starving cougar. Its race-car revving sounded distinctly urgent with a growl that came in waves. The backlit silhouette of a figure was clearly visible in the cab.

'Pony up boy, jump in, switch on, let's skedaddle. Time is of the essence!' the voice shouted over.

Dusty's engine sung, this time accompanied by a wheezing laugh, the sort that spun dirty campfire stories, blew cigarette smoke in your face, and supped from a hip-flask.

Propelled by an unknown force, I ran for the open cabin door and up the steps to ride shotgun. A thick-set cowboy, with long white hair spilling daintily onto his shoulders manned the wheel. Leathery, tattooed skin peeked from under the sleeves of his wildly-embroidered black shirt.

'It's about fuckin' time ya got here, kid,' he said, shooting me a dry grimace. 'We need to get going. Time is tight and only getting tighter. Strap in and let's roll.'

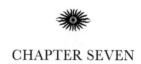

CHAPTER SEVEN

The Gospel of Leuk

When I was diagnosed I had no idea what leukaemia actually was. Not a clue. I had to learn, and fast. I was eager to understand and give context to everything I was undergoing. By learning the medical language spoken all around me, perhaps I could anchor the experience in the facts and statistics of everyday life.

The word leukaemia comes from the Greek *leukos* which means white, and *aima* which means blood. Leukaemia is a form of cancer that causes the bone marrow to produce many more white blood cells than is normal. Fundamentally it is a genetic mutation. Our DNA provides detailed instructions for how each cell should operate. With cancer, certain cells begin to function rather differently in the blood than they should, in my case, aggressively multiplying and crowding out the good guys to the point where they interfere with major bodily organs. This process is called metastasis.

Cancer is a word that everyone has heard of, but a condition few understand. Coined by the 'Father of Medicine', Hippocrates, around 400 BC, cancer has been rampaging through flesh, blood, and bone for as long as humans have been around. The earliest known description was found in ancient Egyptian texts dating from around 3000 BC, where it was declared "there is no treatment".

Cancer doesn't discriminate. It doesn't care about your family, your friends, or your fragile human life. As with so many before me, I instantly gave it form. I personified it as a cruel being, lurking in the bleached-clean shadows of hospital wards, gleefully destroying lives. What else was I to think? All I'd heard was that it was a killer. Something to be truly afraid of. Understandably, I had designated it as evil.

Of course in reality, cancer itself is neither good nor evil, as those are human judgements. It's simply a set of biological processes. A mangled mutation of cells, spiralling out of control. A product of cause and effect onto which we project our own death-born fears, opinions and insecurities.

In the UK at the turn of the millennium, a cancer diagnosis was generally considered a death sentence. I learnt this from a young age through the experiences of friends, family, through the media, and the general zeitgeist surrounding its various forms. We are taught that disease is something external that invades our bodies and can only be cured through extractive treatments, drugs, and probably more drugs. The more we accept this narrative, the more we are disempowered in our own innate healing. The human body's ability to heal itself, and the role of the mind and spirit in matters of disease has been vastly underplayed in the modern age.

We are all aware of the power of placebo, even if we don't yet fully understand it, and can appreciate the difference a positive mindset makes to the outcome of a situation. And yet, many of us struggle with the concept when applying it to 'little old me'.

In the latter half of the 20th century the number of cancer diagnoses rose significantly throughout the west. This correlated with a shift in our dietary and lifestyle choices. In her myth-busting book *The Big Fat Surprise*, Nina Teicholz highlights the marked increase in availability of highly-sugared foods, heavily-processed grains, and the proliferation of cheaply-produced industrial vegetable and seed oils. All of these have in common an ability to dramatically increase inflammation in the body. We now know inflammation to be a leading cause of disease. Consequently such intensive agriculture and it's reliance on toxic pesticides have wreaked havoc on our food supply, degrading the health of our soils, polluting our waters and accelerating species extinction.

Technological gadgets such as the beloved television drew us indoors, slowly severing our connection with the natural world and potentially triggering the breakdown of communities. The rise in cancer diagnoses can also be traced back to the industrial revolution and its insistence that to be of any worth to society we must work extremely long hours in unnatural and detrimental conditions. Before long, high-pressure, productivity-first work environments became the norm, providing the perfect platform for various forms of cancer to thrive. Despite a tsunami of scientific evidence warning us of the mental and physical effects, we are yet to kick the habit.

As technological advancement prolonged the human lifespan, our greatest cultural downfall was solidified: the fear and complete rejection of death. People were living longer, pathogenic diseases became treatable and individuals could focus more on themselves and their own aspirations. With the dawn of individualism, death became enshrined as something we simultaneously feared, despised, and would try to avoid at all costs.

Perhaps there is something more to being alive than just our physical bodies living a singular life, something wider, deeper, and vastly more complex than our waking day-to-day reality. There's a reason Native Americans refer to this concept as The Great Mystery. There are few remaining cultures where death is regarded as a transition into another way of being, something not only accepted but embraced in the social narrative. For our culture, quite the opposite is true. Death defiance is so entrenched that to even contemplate one's own mortality is commonly considered a morbid and decidedly strange thing to do. Why? After all, it is a simple truth that we will die. But we are just not comfortable at the thought of it. Can our discomfort be a marker for what is worthy of deeper enquiry? Are we really living if we are not facing death?

In his 2011 book *The Emperor of All Maladies: A Biography of Cancer*, the oncologist Siddhartha Mukherjee solemnly states that:

> *The arrival of a patient with acute leukaemia still sends a shiver down the hospital's spine—all the way from the cancer wards on its upper floors to the clinical laboratories buried deep in the basement. Leukaemia is a cancer of the white blood cells—cancer in one of*

its most explosive, violent incarnations. As one nurse on the wards often liked to remind her patients, with this disease 'even a paper cut is an emergency.'

He goes on to say that for an oncologist in training, leukaemia represents a special incarnation of cancer:

'Its pace, its acuity, its breathtaking, inexorable arc of growth forces rapid, often drastic decisions; it is terrifying to experience, terrifying to observe, and terrifying to treat. The body invaded by leukaemia is pushed to its brittle physiological limit—every system, heart, lung, blood, working at the knife-edge of its performance.'

There are both chronic and acute forms of leukaemia. Diagnosis will find you assigned to one of these two groups. In its most simplistic terms, these groupings describe how quickly the leukaemia is likely to develop and worsen. They are then sub-grouped into which kind of blood cells are affected.

Acute leukaemias develop rapidly and can become life-threatening very quickly, while chronic leukaemias are the opposite – they develop slowly and tend to get worse over long periods of time. In chronic leukaemias – which generally affect adults over the age of fifty-five – the white blood cells are almost, but not completely, normal. They still function to a degree, but not as well as they should in fighting and removing external infections. With acute leukaemias – which tend to target younger people and children – large numbers of white blood cells are prematurely released. These are known as blast cells and are much less effective at fighting infections.

Topping the blood cell hierarchy are stem cells – blank templates from which all other blood cells are made. From here two lineages are created. Myeloid stem cells in the bone marrow are precursors to red blood cells, platelets and others. Lymphoid cells develop into T-cells, B-cells and natural killer cells, and are related to the lymphatic system, an integral part of our immunity.

Lymphoid cancers are termed 'lymphoblastic', and myeloid simply 'myeloid.' The vast majority of people diagnosed with acute leukaemia, as I was, either have acute lymphoblastic leukaemia (ALL) or acute myeloid leukaemia (AML). Generally, young adults and children are diagnosed with ALL, whilst in older folks, there is a trend towards AML.

My diagnosis was kind of neither. It was acute undifferentiated leukaemia (AUL). This is the name they give to all the various non-myeloid leukaemias, so-called because they usually feature the diagnostic markers of both ALL and AML, but can sometimes have no markers of either. Consequently, I became something of a minor celebrity on my ward: the boy with the rare blood cancer. Less than 1% of cases have this classification.

My course of treatment would now have to be tailored to this condition, which basically meant they had to treat these rogue lymphoid markers too. The next round of chemotherapy would consist of the two main drugs intended to treat the myeloid element, mitoxantrone and high dose cytosine. Then at the start of each week's treatment, I would also get a dose of vinchristine and prednisolone, a combination to induce apoptosis – the programmed death of cancer cells. If all of that wasn't enough, Doc Oc was worried about the lymphoid markers affecting the area around my brain, so he was also giving me a substance with the delightfully murderous name of methotrexate. Unlike the others, this immunosuppressant would be injected directly into my spinal canal so it could reach my cerebrospinal fluid undisturbed. If that all sounds like overkill, that's because quite literally, it is.

According to Cancer Research UK, leukaemia is the tenth most common cancer among males in the UK, with almost six-thousand new cases annually. Although over 73% of men survive for at least a year, sadly only 53% of us make it to five years. 41% of us mark a decade. These are the latest 2017 statistics. When my treatment began back in 1999, survival rates were around 40% for a five year period, with 30% reaching ten years. The odds of surviving long-term were evidently not in my favour.

Our bodies are home to various types of T-cells (Thymus-dependent lymphocytes). These workhorses of the immune system regulate its activity. Cytotoxic T-cells target cancerous cells and pathogens, whether they are bacterial or viral in origin. But to eliminate certain infections undetectable to T-cells, a ruthless lymphocyte known as natural killer (NK) cells are needed. They were first recognised for their distinct ability to destroy tumour cells without any prior priming or activation. These guys are the contract killers of our blood. Researchers are currently developing immunotherapy treatments involving the programming of NK cells for specific tasks.

During my illness, I could feel my body struggle. I'd even go so far as to say that I could feel my immune cells fighting as my entire system tried to haul itself back from the precipice of defeat. As symptoms flared and blood pulsed around my body, the steady rise and fall of my breathing took my attention inward.

A biological battle was happening and it was real. It wasn't under my direct control, yet my immune system fought with incredible intensity around the clock. These inner actions were palpable and instinctively my desire was to fan those flames, to fuel each and every part of me with absolute will and determination. All my mental and physical energy was given over to the processes my body was entrenched in. Be it intuition, character or innate reflex, I chose to actively engage with my inner biology.

I understood that a positive mindset would boost my chances. The new science of psychoneuroimmunology bears this out. Research shows that self-belief and the cultivation of a positive mindset directly affects the response of our immune system. Put simply, our attitude has a definite impact on the outcome of our treatment. The mechanics of this are clarified by Patricia Peat in her excellent guide to cancer treatment, *The Cancer Revolution*:

> *'This field was spearheaded by Dr Candace Pert (1948-2013) and colleagues in the 1990s in Molecules of Emotion, which proved that our emotions profoundly affect our body chemistry, immune systems and the functioning of all body tissues. This science shows that communication within the body is not just coming to and from our brains, but that all of our cells make and receive messages via 'informational substances' known as neuropeptides. If we are sad, depressed, stressed and emotionally repressed, our tissue functioning also becomes depressed. Most critically, in cancer, this*

*means that cells lose their innate protection mechanisms and also
that our immune function depletes, resulting in there being fewer
white blood cells that are aggressive in nature, with a lower number
of the all-important NK cells that can detect and kill cancer cells.'*

The suggestion of positive thinking during a crisis has long
been a divisive one. It can be harmfully dismissive and create barriers when accessing support. Clearly there is more to this than
reaching for rose-tinted glasses. In one of my all-time favourite
books, *Healing and The Mind*, Bill Moyers explores the mind-body
connection through a series of long-form interviews with experts
across a variety of fields. From this fascinating collection, a quote
by Dr. Candace Pert stood out:

*'A common ingredient in the healing practices of native cultures
is catharsis, complete release of emotion. Positive thinking is
interesting, but if it denies the truth, I can't believe that would
anything except bad.'*

I think what Pert is referring to is what's known as 'toxic positivity', a type of bypassing common within spiritual circles, which
ignores the reality of a situation in the hope of manifesting an entirely
new one. This is very different to the benefits of acknowledging
the struggle, finding things to be grateful for and having hope of
better days to come – striving for positive change over pretending
we are waving not drowning.

Being optimistic is a gamble. Studies have shown that it can set
one up for failure if there are expectations of a certain outcome.

The eternal optimist who cannot stop fighting might actually cause greater stress on their body than those who understand the importance of strategic retreat in a complicated long-term process. Allowing yourself to recuperate is as valuable as seizing the moment to swing your sword

Chemotherapy is one of the most infamously toxic substances used in western medicine. It is the cumulative name given to a family of over one hundred extremely high strength drugs. Pumped into the veins in liquid form, they traverse the body via the blood, treating cancer cells wherever they hide. Chemo can be applied to many different forms of cancer, killing cells that are in the process of dividing. This is what makes it so effective.

Cancer cells multiply at a much faster rate than normal cells, making them a recognisable target. Some kill the cells at the point of splitting, while others work by impairing genes inside a cell's nucleus, the control centre that governs their behaviour, therefore disrupting the key processes that allow for cell division. Problems arise because the chemo is incapable of differentiating between regular and cancerous cells. Our hair is always growing, our skin and digestive lining constantly renew, and our bone marrow, the very seedbed of the blood, is continuously regenerating. Unavoidably, healthy cells are sacrificed.

During chemotherapy the body is subjected to a highly traumatic experience and a whole host of side-effects can occur. Nausea and sickness, diarrhoea, gastric upset, hair loss, brain fog, mobility issues, appetite loss, and hearing loss are the most common. Usually, the body can replace or repair damaged cells, and once treatment is complete the acute effects typically ease off. Chemo is well-known for it's potential long-term issues – infertility, early onset menopause, improper functioning of the heart, liver, kidneys, and lungs as well as nerve damage, especially to the hands and feet.

Immune cells in the blood are also impacted, reducing the body's ability to fight infection. Platelets diminish too, these are the cells that are responsible for blood clotting. For those with very low numbers such as haemophiliacs, a simple paper cut can be fatal if not treated. Platelets are strange things. Arriving at my bedside as a floppy plastic pouch of yellow-orange jelly, before dripping into my bloodstream through the Hickman line. I received many bags of them.

With my white blood cells behaving so erratically, chemo was my only real chance. When you're given two weeks to live there's no time to ponder over interventional diets or jet off to the jungles of Peru for a few rounds of desperately intensive plant medicine. Credit where it's due – one of the strengths of western medicine most definitely lies in swiftly performing extreme interventions; in my case, that was exactly what was needed.

How well conventional cancer treatments do mostly depends on what kind of cancer you have, the severity, and the spread of those cells. Even if chemotherapy is unlikely to provide a lasting cure, it is the go-to for doctors to shrink tumours, relieve symptoms, and take control of the cancer. Their goal, as far as I understand it, is remission.

If you are said to be 'in remission', it means that cancer is currently undetectable in the body. Partial remission, however, means some cancer cells are still detectable but are not seen to be growing any further. Cancer cells are clever and are known to hide within organs and the spinal fluid. This is why the best chance of a full remission, especially with an aggressive blood cancer such as mine, is through a bone marrow transplant (BMT).

Since my hospitalisation twenty-two years ago, I've read that treatments have improved and medical knowledge has evolved, allowing for faster and more accurate diagnosis. The same side-effects remain, although the anecdotal evidence from patients using cannabis to mitigate nausea and appetite-suppression is encouraging.

The antioxidant compound N-Acetyl Cysteine (NAC) has received much attention online in the past few years, with articles listing the multifunctional benefits of this well-researched and low-cost supplement. It is promoted as a protector and detoxifier of the liver and kidneys, as well as treating psychiatric disorders and addictive behaviours.

Studies at Mansoura University, Egypt, have also shown NAC to mitigate some chemo side-effects in children with ALL or Lymphoma, when combined with Vitamin E. Interestingly, researchers at the University of Salford, UK, observed NAC inhibiting the protein responsible for tumour growth in breast cancer patients. The jury is still out on it's use in oncology, however, as it may reduce the anti-tumour effects of chemotherapy. Nevertheless, this readily-available compound is well worth looking into, and I believe it to be a valuable addition to the medicine cabinet.

Personally, I use NAC as a liver protector prior to social situations in which I might indulge in alcoholic drinks. Due to my adult-onset asthma, I also use it for its ability to repair damaged lung tissue and as an mucolytic – a substance which breaks down mucous in the lungs.

A ground-breaking approach in the evolution of cancer treatment comes in the form of an experimental immunotherapy known as CAR-T. Chimeric Antigen Receptor T-cell therapy is designed to strengthen the body's natural defences against cancer. Extracting and genetically engineering the patient's own T-cells, makes them better able to recognise and eliminate cancer cells. After being grown in the lab, they are then placed back into the patient's bloodstream, usually after a round of chemotherapy. They remain in the body as a 'living drug' for some time afterwards to guard against a possible return. It sounds wildly futuristic but it is now becoming a reality.

Until recently, the use of CAR-T has been restricted to small-scale trials involving patients with advanced blood cancers, delivering remarkable results in those for whom all other treatments have failed. At the time of writing, CAR-T has been successfully trialled in children with ALL, and promisingly the NHS have announced they'll be offering it for selected cases of ALL and Diffuse large B-cell lymphoma in the UK. Research is ongoing but the belief is the therapy could also be engineered to target tumours using NK cells in the future. This method heralds a revolution in the way such diseases are treated, with the potential to all together remove the need for bone marrow or stem cell transplants.

Cancer cells are effectively on a suicide mission. They have no fear of dying, only a drive for disabling the system – the careless anarchist, violently rejecting normality for the sake of it, biting the hand that feeds them. In most other illnesses, the body tries to prevent pathogenic invaders from making it their weakened host. So when disruption is an internal affair, the surrounding cells stand by in disbelief as numbers of their own join the coup. A once harmonious network falls into chaos as this ragtag gang, working independently under the guise of a team, focus only on proliferation. Without intervention, they will kill the host. Nihilistic little buggers, yet they are not separate from us. My cancer cells were still a part of me. I wanted to reach them, to start a dialogue; to find out why they took this path of corruption and discover how they could be stopped.

Strangely, no-one really knows what triggers the different kinds of leukaemia in most cases, why our blood cells suddenly behave in this abnormal way. From the data so far, scientists conclude that it develops under a combination of lifestyle, genetic and environmental conditions. There are many theories involving mobile phones, powerlines and pesticides, but currently little evidence to support them. Verified factors that elevate a person's risk of blood cancer include: compromised immunity, viruses, post-chemo medication, exposure to EMF, house paint, and a chemical known as benzene used in the industrial production of shoes, rubber, pharmaceuticals and petrol. Traffic pollution has also been indicated.

Possibly one of the most significant risk factors is ionising radiation exposure. It has the potential to damage our DNA, yet is widely used within diagnostic medicine and global energy production. My mother maintains that multiple X-Rays during her first trimester activated my leukaemia. After her initial procedure, she recalls having a strong negative response. When doctors insisted on further scans, she refused, but was later coaxed into it against her better judgement. There may well be something to that, but it's also natural for a mother to find cause within her own actions.

Environmental exposure to non-ionising radiation has also been implicated in leukaemia cases. My family home was two doors down from an electrical substation, a small fenced compound which delivered electricity to the neighbourhood. Could this EMF have contributed to my diagnosis? It's plausible. In 2015, the European Commission Scientific Committee on Emerging and Newly Identified Health Risks concluded that 'extremely low frequency fields show an increased risk of childhood leukaemia.' This is especially alarming when considering the prevalence of smart devices in children's everyday lives.

We all know that smoking causes cancer, graphic images of tumours are plastered across every cigarette packet, yet little is ever said about how it puts adults at greater risk of developing acute myeloid leukaemia. Smoking doesn't just affect the individual. The study *Parental Smoking and the Risk of Childhood Leukemia*, published by Jeffrey S. Chang et al. in the *American Journal of Epidemiology*, states results 'strongly suggests that exposure to paternal preconception smoking alone or in combination with postnatal passive smoking may be important in the risk of childhood leukemia.' I don't believe smoking played a significant role in my story but allow me to reiterate what struck me most about this risk – men who smoke carry the possibility of leukaemia within their sperm. Hopefully this contributes to raising awareness.

Up until 2018, leukaemia posed a terrifying threat to lives without anyone knowing how to prevent it. Then, after three decades of studying childhood leukaemia, a scientist by the name of Mel Greaves, based at the Institute of Cancer Research in London, discovered a pattern. Driven by his obsession to understand why these young patients developed the disease, he noticed that it was more prevalent amongst developed societies than developing ones. Greaves found leukaemia tracks with affluence, increasing in the UK and Europe at the rate of 1% a year.

Acute lymphoblastic leukaemia is caused by a two-pronged sequence of genetic mutations. In other words, two provoking events are needed. The first occurs in about one in twenty children, caused by an incident in the womb. The second involves immunity. When a child's health is over-shielded in the first year of life their immune system is denied vital opportunities to develop. Without being sufficiently primed, it can overreact to later infections, causing chronic inflammation. In response, cytokines are released into the blood stream, triggering the second mutation in the sequence. Children who carry both mutations are at genuine risk of developing the disease. It is an extremely worrying scenario that in our quest for longevity, our modern-day obsession with cleanliness, the steady spread of anti-bacterial products and the demonisation of dirt, we may actually be putting our children in danger.

Hope comes in the form of Dr Greaves' understanding of the potential power within our microbiome, the colonies of bacteria and other microbes that live in the gut. With experts paying closer attention to the microscopic inhabitants of our digestive system, we've learned how a greater diversity of bacteria leads to better immunity – up to 80% of the body's immune cells are located in the gut.

Dr Greaves and his team are now working to highlight specific bacterias with immune-stimulating properties. Their plan is to produce a yogurt-like drink for very young children, with the aim of preventing the second mutation from occurring, dramatically lowering the risk of childhood leukaemia. Human trials are expected within two to three years. Probiotic soft drinks such as kefir and kombucha, once the preserve of underground folk tales, can now be found on the shelves of major supermarket chains as people wake up to the benefits of regularly consuming fermented foods.

Not all that long ago, pickles, preserves and ferments were commonplace in the home – cheap and nutritious staples. Flashy adverts for branded food and goods pushed out the homemade and handcrafted in favour of a modern lifestyle. Perhaps unsurprisingly, ferments have risen in profile in recent years, their many benefits now lauded by companies rushing to jump on the bandwagon. It seems to be the way of things – great changes often start on the fringes and steadily seep into the mainstream over time, as if by osmosis.

The high fat, low-carb, ketogenic diet has exploded in popularity over the last few years. People are adopting this way of eating to address excess weight, to maintain physical and mental energy, overcome metabolic diseases, improve their athletic performance, make their brains work better, and to control seizures. While it may not be the best approach for everybody – especially long-term – for some it appears to be very useful.

More and more medical practitioners are prescribing the 'keto diet', and researchers are exploring its utility in the treatment and prevention of cancer. The primary benefit for an oncology patient is that ketosis – a metabolic state where fat becomes the primary fuel source – can potentially enhance a cancer cell's susceptibility to chemo whilst normal cells are better protected.

After my treatment, I was left with a weakened immune system and a gut microbiome that had been deeply damaged by litres of chemotherapy and bags of antibiotics. With little help from the medical establishment, I had to experiment and rebuild it from scratch. Fermented foods and holistic nutrition played an important role in that process. They continue to be a cornerstone of my health strategy, inspired by Functional Medicine – a biology-based approach that focuses on identifying and addressing the root cause of disease.

It truly lifts me to hear of patients and families taking an active role in their treatment and recovery. There is a burgeoning movement, primarily internet-led, of people choosing to incorporate highly-potent, full-spectrum preparations of a plant that is presently illegal in the UK. *Cannabis sativa* is possibly one of the most under-appreciated and misrepresented medicinal allies – as I briefly mentioned earlier, cannabis has been seen to ease certain side-effects of chemotherapy.

Of the most well-known cannabinoids, Tetrahydrocannabinol (THC) is cited in the successful breakdown of tumours, while Cannabidiol (CBD) has proved effective at managing pain, anxiety and muscular spasms. Some people even report the reversal of

Stage Four conditions, where the cancer has spread to other parts of the body and formed secondary cancers, much to the surprise of their doctors.

Our body's ability to make use of cannabinoids is via a complex signalling network known as the endocannabinoid system (ECS). This plays an important role in the modulation of immunity, inflammation, pain and stress, as well as vital body systems. Although other plants can stimulate its two main receptors – known as CB1 and CB2 – cannabis is the most effective. Experts are currently engaged in multiple studies to fully understand its workings, but maintaining homeostasis appears to be its primary function.

As science catches up with the profound subtleties of the ECS, the popular Facebook groups *C.K.C (Cannabis Kills Cancer)* and *Cannabis Oil Success Stories* are buzzing with pioneering individuals documenting their own experiential cannabis protocols. Another resource I find fascinating is the *Cannabis Health Radio* podcast, which presents personal stories of healing across hundreds of episodes. They lend weight to the wave of research that seeks to re-establish cannabis as a powerful medicine; a natural approach to the prevention, treatment and symptom-management of cancer.

I believe we're moving towards a future where cannabis-based therapies, alongside the groundbreaking CAR-T and new forms of targeted immunotherapy, provide a winning combination. It's exciting and heart-warming to observe the approaches to treating this frightening disease evolving right before our very eyes.

Ω

Time is Tight

The cowboy rammed his boot to the floor and we lurched away, spitting up stones, a cloud of dust billowing up behind us. I glanced over at the old man who turned to me and winked, one hand on the wheel, the other resting out the window. His wrinkled face was calm, the edges of his mouth slightly upturned. The sun blazed through his lank white hair, confessing untold stories. On his head, sat a timeless black stetson, its aged threads starting to fail.

'Sorry to bust your chops like that, its jus' that time is my trade. We got places to do and things to be y'know?'

'No it's, er... fine.'

'Real good of you to join me on this trip. Real good.'

He chuckled to himself and began humming Cream's 'Sunshine of Your Love', tapping out its loping rhythm with panache on the pale leather steering wheel. The bus filled with Ginger Baker's

wild toms. The cowboy looo-ooiyoh-oh-iyohoove'd along with
Jack Bruce at the top of his voice. Faster we went, and I saw there
was no speedometer on the dashboard, no instrument panel of
any kind. Surely we were going faster than this dust-bucket could
handle? The barren landscape became a blur as the music carried
us up and onwards in its hypnotic swirl.

Being around him gave me a strong sense of deja vu, as if we'd
met before. It didn't cross my mind to question his intent because
getting into a strange American man's Winnebago in the middle of
the desert had seemed perfectly normal, almost as if I was expecting it.

'I'm sorry, but I'm a bit confused. Where are we going?'

'Ask the mountain, kid. Right now I'm in need of sustenance.
Then we got hay to make.'

Without loading a disc or pressing any buttons, the sound of
Jimi Hendrix, live and high on LSD flooded the space, that classic
guitar tone cranking out from every surface, as if the whole vehicle
was at once the source and the speakers.

We sped on through the wide lunar expanse, following the sun
westwards, leaving the dunes far behind. The mountains were clearly
visible now and consequently the landscape was changing. Trees
and grasses started to appear, and ahead on a hillside, a smattering
of glowing orange dots signified a settlement. As we got nearer the
shimmering lights morphed into houses. My driver swung the bus
round into the picket-fenced parking lot of a tumbledown diner at
the far end of town. A failing neon hoarding announced, through
frazzled flashes, that this was 'Debbie's Place' and that we were
most welcome. No other vehicles occupied the empty bays. Had
my attention not been stolen by the hunchback shadow shuffling

around inside like a mammoth in an apron, I'd have assumed the place was long since deserted, devoid of all life.

Cutting a rather fine figure in his crisp shirt and faded denim, the cowboy led the way. Pushing open the swinging double doors, he wandered past the rusting bar stools, settling his frame into a red leather booth. I followed suit.

The hunched monster I'd seen silhouetted against the gloom of the counter was actually human. She was a beast of a woman, seven feet tall at least with mound upon mound of fatty rolls. Her ridiculously tight top struggled to contain her and she stunk of rotting vegetables.

The cowboy coughed deliberately, alerting her to our presence. Startled, she looked up in disbelief at the strangers who dared enter her domain. Her mood soured.

'Two house burgers with everything, please my sweet,' asked the cowboy, turning on the charm, 'and my, don't you look lovely today.' He flashed his pearly-whites, curiously immaculate for someone of his lifestyle and advancing years.

'Huhha, yuh. Furruh puhhn,' Debbie frothed. A hail of saliva sprayed from her mouth as she waddled over, surely intent on violently crushing the life out of her sole patrons, groaning more unintelligible phrases.

Before reaching the end of the bar she suddenly stopped in her tracks, silent, head cocked at an angle as if listening to something only she was privy to hear. Seconds ticked by. Then, as if nothing had happened, our waitress trotted off to the kitchen. A clatter of pots and pans could be heard above occasional grunts, seemingly her favoured form of communication.

Debbie was frightening but I sympathised. All cooped up in the middle of nowhere on her own, condemned to shuffle around a deteriorating restaurant, scowling at the rats, devouring anything she could lay her filthy hands on. Stringy cobwebs hung from the ceiling and coffee spills had stained the chequered vinyl floor. The age of the decor and its slow descent into decay was partially obscured in the half-light, but the thick layer of dust and grime coating our table told me that no-one had dined here in a very long time.

'You must be hungry, journey you've been on,' said the cowboy, apparently unfazed by the surroundings.

'I'm not sure... I guess I'll eat if you are?'

'Yeah, you should eat.'

Seconds later, the giantess re-emerged. Sweat streamed from her brow in shallow tributaries, her lifeless hair plastered across her forehead. She dropped two great white plates down in front of us, sounding her irritation. Heading for a dark corner, she slumped down on the floor and began picking her nose, searching for the ripest specimens.

Surprisingly, the burger was the most incredible I'd ever seen: bacon, melted cheese, sliced tomato, crispy lettuce, zingy relish, dripping fried egg, juicy pineapple, and lashings of mayonnaise topped the double patties. Even the sesame-seed bun had been warmed. We tucked in with vigour. The cowboy demolished his before I'd even taken a second bite of mine. With the back of his hand he wiped the juice from his chin.

'That's what I call a meal!' he announced, slapping his thigh with gusto, 'eat up, young buck, you'll be needing all your strength soon enough.'

I gladly obliged, leaving nothing but a plate of crumbs and a few strips of wilted lettuce.

'That's what I'm talking about,' he said, reaching for his stetson. 'Now we really should beat feet. Ya can't waste time.'

'But I've only just finished eating, I don't think I can move yet,' I protested.

'Don't think, jus' do. That's my motto. I swear by it, how it's been my whole damn existence. Truth be told, it's seen me through the darkest of days, I can tell you, son. I get up and I keep going and ain't nothin' gonna stop me, hah!' He raised his palm to offer a wrinkled high-five, which I readily accepted.

CHAPTER EIGHT

Freedom

My parents had responded with defiant dedication to the seismic shift in our family life.

After a month off, Dad went back to work. He would finish teaching around half-past three, jump in the car and drive the forty miles or so from Wolverhampton, where he was Head of Maths, to Shrewsbury Hospital, keep me company for a couple of hours, before arriving back in Bridgnorth tired and hungry at around 8 pm. Mum and Dad would try to unwind over a glass of wine as they talked about the latest news, what aspects of my treatment they were going to research next and how they were both coping.

They moved heaven and earth to keep their visits consistent. Their full-time teaching careers had suddenly become the least important thing in their lives – a hindrance to their need to be with me. They alternated after-work visits, juggling the day-to-day problems of the other siblings and care of Mac the dog.

It was essential to the collective family mindset to keep things going. My parents worked hard to retain a base level of normality. Brave faces were slapped on in response to the many questions from worried friends and neighbours. Sustaining this for my siblings was a constant effort. When Dad had explained to my headteacher that I was critically ill with leukaemia, asking him to place my academic life on pause, he fought back tears, made his excuses and quickly left.

Doc Oc and the nursing team had been monitoring my stats religiously: temperature, blood pressure, blood counts, and the rest of the endlessly fluctuating levels. I always made sure to ask for a detailed update from the doctor himself.

I found myself analysing the process too, studying my appearance, looking in the mirror a little longer each time I went to the bathroom. Observing my body as it shifted before my eyes. Was my skin beginning to change colour? I was both afraid and fascinated at my reflection. I felt as if I could almost see the drugs moving around. My sallow face, sunken eyes and cheekbones, all the more prominent now, looked back with a doleful gaze. I'd built such strong legs biking uphill for a paper-round job, and now my thighs resembled those of a scrawny child.

The scared boy in the mirror had eyes that were darker than I remembered, his skin translucent and pallid. I told him: this was not a done deal. Not at all. This was just the way things were right now. It was shitty, but if we wanted out of this strange dream, then my past and present selves would have to get on board. This didn't need to be a death sentence.

For several mornings, I woke to find clumps of hair strewn across my starched white pillow. I'd been told to expect it but nothing can prepare you for the bizarre experience of your hair lazily falling away from your head like feathers on the breeze. After a couple of days, they asked me if I'd like it all shaved off. I thankfully accepted. A male nurse turned up armed with battered clippers and expertly buzzed me clean – obviously well-practiced.

The thick covering of hair on my arms and legs rinsed off with the shower gel. I'd find bundles of stray pubes hanging out in my boxers each time I went to the loo. I felt like a plucked chicken with a severe case of eczema. Dry and flaky, my body was deteriorating under the pressure. Slowly but surely the chemotherapy was going about its dark work. I had completed my transformation into the stereotypical teenage cancer patient; I could have been a poster boy for leukaemia.

I hated what the drugs were doing to me and the acute side effects were depressing to accept. I felt like key aspects of what made me *me* had been eroded. I wondered if I'd ever get them back.

To help bolster my mental attitude through all this hardship, I fervently dreamt about life post-cancer; here I have tattoos, go to music festivals and experiment with drugs, discover faraway lands and other cultures, and live out my new-found love with Tash. In this future I enjoy a life of purpose.

Such hopes had been brought into sharp focus a week into my treatment, when Doc Oc realised he'd forgotten to take any semen samples before beginning chemo. If I was to have children at some point in the future, IVF would be the only way my genes could be part of the process. Given that my treatment was almost certain to result in infertility, this delay in salvaging my swimmers added to my mental load.

Assuring us there was still time, the apologetic Luanne delivered a small pot to my room. She empathised, knowing very well the state I'd been in over the previous few days – providing a semen sample would be an exceptionally tall order. Somehow, many minutes later, I managed to dispense the required amount. It came out looking tired and pale... even my spunk was depressed.

Despite the failings of my body, my mind was still sharp. I had taken a real interest in the atomic workings of the disease and every aspect of my treatment. I gained unique first-hand insights, and at times felt I probably knew more than the squeaky-clean junior doctors who traipsed nervously after Doc Oc as he made his twice-daily rounds.

It was my body. It seemed only natural to want to know every detail about the drugs, how they would act and what trials I would be put through. I urged them to tell the whole truth and let me digest it face-to-face. I deeply valued knowing the score and being fully aware of all the likely possibilities. It was always a case of, 'Right, what's next? What is the next stage? Where do we go now?' My questions often put them on the spot, and to his credit, Doc Oc encouraged this. For him, it was a definite positive sign to see a patient so actively engaged with overcoming their predicament, to the extent of learning the medical terms and their meanings.

Why should I have to take 10mg of powdered potassium in a plastic water cup that tastes like drinking seawater? *Because chemotherapy can cause your kidneys to excrete more potassium than they usually would.* How long would it take for my white blood cell count to come back? *It all depended on the speed at which your immune system could recover.* When would this prednisolone stop making me feel like a piece of discarded chewing gum, its flavour ground down, spat out onto the pavement for any passersby to step on? *Once the drugs are stopped, so are the side-effects.*

Shooting pains at breakfast, followed by wretching at lunch and leg cramps before dinner. Sometime after that, my meal re-appeared. After another two weeks of intermittent diarrhoea, vomiting, mouth sores, loss of appetite and vitality, my body began the uphill struggle to claw back control once more.

A few days later the regular sickness settled somewhat and I was able to keep down a small meal. My white cells started to grow again, break out into my bloodstream and generate the all-important neutrofils. When my white cell count reached above 8.0 and my neutrofils 2.0, I was permitted another leave of absence, to return home to family dinners and evenings happily watching TV together.

A third and final round of chemo awaited me upon my return but six full days of freedom were mine. I longed to inhale something other than disinfectant and the cloying odour of my own stinking sweat and vomit. The artificial cleanliness of my environment destroyed any sense of comfort. At home, I could relax, take a long soak in the bath, and try to work up the strength to go through the whole thing once more.

Again, I was warned not to touch any alcohol, salads, cream-cheese and all the other culinary no-no's. I would have to avoid crowds, public places, and people with even the slightest of sniffles. Bacteria and infection were the greatest threats. My immunity had been seriously compromised by the treatments and I had to be handled gently, treated with almost as much care as a newborn child, a pregnant mother, or the very elderly.

Most of all, I looked forward to spending some precious alone time with Tasha. It was bound to be weird to begin with, but all I wanted, even more than Mum's Sunday roast, was to curl up on a bed with her in my arms and feel like some kind of a man again, to forget the boy in the mirror.

Our relationship had held strong through the first stages of my illness. Her hand in mine and a few lingering hugs were about as much contact as we had gotten. Tash generally sat on my bed or beside me during her visits. Now, I craved the full warmth of her naked body for the first time in weeks. I needed to hold her and silently show just how much her love and support meant to me. Aside from my parents, she was the only force outside of myself that was able to drive me onwards.

Sadly my libido had been shot to pieces and even if by some miracle I could have got it up, the doctors had said sex was out of the question. Too much of a risk for one so weak inside.

Waking to bright clear sunshine, I politely refused the stand-ard-issue breakfast offered by a smiling Luanne, explaining that Mum had taken the day off work to treat me to a slap-up brunch in Shrewsbury. We'd agreed on it the week before, a little celebration to mark the end of the second chemo cycle, to provide some sense of normalcy. Whatever I fancied in the restaurant was mine to choose.

I showered and dressed with what little vigour I could muster.

A slight spring was detectable in my step, perhaps the result of my white blood cells slowly multiplying and the thrill of revisiting simplicities I once took for granted.

Outside, the late-November frost had cast a white sheen over the grassy banks of the hospital grounds, right across the yellowing trees, bronzed with dying autumnal hues, to the recesses of the main car park. It was a brave new world out there. I imagined the cold air whipping at my face as I breathed in life. Hopefully, Mum had remembered to pack my black woolly gloves, old fleece scarf, and my reliable grey duffle coat as instructed, or it would be a treacherous walk to the car.

The heating in my room was cranked up, keeping me toasty as I lay back on the bed, sipping a tea, watching a riveting cooking challenge. I soon tired of the TV and flicked on the stereo – something upbeat would put me in the right mood. On her last visit, Tasha had brought along a few CDs she knew I'd love, and thoughtfully, a brand new O'Neill beanie to warm my bare head. By this point I'd played my Feeder record to death, but still, its comforting sing-along rock was all I wanted to hear. I pressed play, careful not to have the volume too loud and risk another motherly ticking-off from Mary.

As the clock showed almost thirty minutes past nine, Mum appeared at my door, her cheeks flushed pink with cold, keen to wrap her arms around her son and grateful to see a smile on his face. Luanne dropped by to chat about my latest progress, blood counts, and charts. Spending some time deliberating over whether I was allowed to eat cucumber with the skin on, they revised the conditions of my release; foods to avoid and situations to steer clear of. Of course, it was decided that safe was better than sorry. Luanne handed Mum a full list of everything to avoid for safe-keeping

Bags all packed full of clothes and carriers bulging with protein shakes and four large bottles of pills, I was set to go. I beamed from ear to ear, waving goodbye to both nurses who waved back.

'No sex, drugs or rock 'n roll please!' hollered Mary with a mischievous grin.

'Watch out for those cucumbers!' winked Luanne. 'See you on Saturday, around six is fine.'

Freedom. Out from those four fucking walls and into the shoes of liberation. Out of the pale ward that housed my room, and through a succession of peach-licked corridors, another hospital colour scheme success. We rode the lift down until the big front doors were in sight. Walking slowly, my aching and underused muscles were not ready for the leaps and bounds that my heart felt like doing – a Dick Van Dyke dance along the walkway to the car.

I was quiet and attentive on the short journey to the city centre. I remember gazing upon the world with a new fascination as the ever-changing fields full of uninterested cattle stared back at me. My eyes viewed the world with a freshness I'd never experienced before. To anyone else, the sight of a cow navigating the hardened mud of a frosty field wouldn't make much of a lasting impression, but to me, this signalled life was still moving forward. Trees were still growing, people were still making it through each day, filling themselves with new thoughts and ideas and navigating the ups and downs of life. My problems became but a minnow in a sea of a million fish: nothing that special.

This heightened perception lingered as we entered a rustic,

converted townhouse by the River Severn. It was just after ten, not the busiest time of day. A few people stood at the bar while around a third of the tables were occupied. A small fire roared away at one end of the room. I ordered bacon and egg, tomatoes and mushrooms, and hash browns. The fullest full English they would serve. My appetite was still yo-yo-ing, but I was determined to give this my best shot. The various aromas wafting out from the kitchen made my stomach grumble with delight. I caught Mum smiling at me as I gazed longingly at the menu. I grinned back, happy for the change of environment.

All I wanted was real food, warmth, and comfort. Anything else was secondary. Mum was going to fuss over me, cooking great meals. Dad would rent a selection of films from the local video store. My kind siblings would make me sympathetic mugs of tea and bring me bags of sweets bought on their way home from school. I was naturally going to be the centre of everyone's attention. Again, I was reminded of how lucky I was to have such a caring home life to go back to.

I managed just over half of the breakfast before giving up in manful recognition of defeat. We spent most of the meal talking about my treatments, the progress, and the next steps. I was getting a bit fed up of hearing about it. Just for a few days, I wanted to forget the gathering clouds on the horizon and simply soak up the moment.

I fell asleep in the car on the journey back, waking just as we swung a tight corner. Passing my school, I gazed up at the red-brick buildings, visualising Tasha in the art studios creating a masterpiece. I thought to reach her with my mind. Concentrating hard, I pinched my eyes, determined to send her my love. As if in response, the rectangular lump in my jean pocket vibrated, causing my leg to shudder.

> **From:** Tash
> **Sent:** 13:41 pm
> Freedoooooom! You busy this week then sailor?
> Can't wait to squeeze you :) T xxx

My heart floated up in my chest and a burning heat surrounded my head. Soon I'd be holding her close, breathing her in. I couldn't wait to bury my face in her tussled blonde hair and stare into those feline eyes. Just taking her all in. I swore to remember every second of it, to record each precious moment in my mind. When things got so hard that I didn't know how I was going to continue, thoughts of her were all I could hold onto to get me through another grey and aching day.

The first meal back home was memorable. We all sat around the big wooden dining table, its scuffs and dinks marking the many times we'd shared stories over Mum's amazing cooking. I grinned at the sight of our family – together again. Home-cooked dinners felt like the height of luxury compared to the lukewarm plates which passed for food at the hospital. Black and white portraits of great-great-grandparents and other relatives watched over us with their stern, unwavering expressions, as if conveying the difficulties of their nineteenth-century lives. I wondered if anyone ever smiled back then.

Outside through the patio door, the garden looked calm,

bathed in peaceful darkness. I almost felt like an intruder in my own home. Oblivious to all the comings and goings and daily events that had taken place there in the last month, I realised I was completely out of touch with their lives. People only ever asked me questions, I hadn't had the ability to ask any of my own; to hear how everyone else was coping. My body was too busy dealing with its primary task, interest in their lives had become completely secondary to my own. I thought about this over a mouthful of Mum's treacle tart.

The next day I'd arranged to stay at Tash's place. I loved going round there – it was quirky and full of delights, from her dad's music room in the basement, complete with a top-of-the-range Naim Hi-Fi setup, to the sound of the birds and the constant delicate trickle of the brook outside her bedroom window. We ate slightly burnt pizza and cuddled up in bed, watching films and kissing gently as night fell.

We awoke in the late morning, folded in each other's arms. Breakfast was juicy bacon and egg sandwiches. In the afternoon we played board games badly and giggled at the latest school gossip. It felt like a seductive dream, a fleeting vision of how my life could one day unfold. I had only four days left before heading back for the third round of treatment and decided to postpone any thoughts of the future until it was right there in front of me. I found happiness in these simple moments and for now that was all I wanted to focus on.

Gradually, my smile returned in earnest and I began to recognise embers of inner strength gently smouldering inside. It gave me hope, the bravery to think of a future in which I'd beaten the disease. I swore to myself, I would do all the things I had ever wanted to, not letting anything stand in my way.

I ate like a king for those six glorious days, fattening myself up in preparation for another few weeks where the best thing I could hope to taste was the acidic bile of my stomach contents. Mealtimes were spent pinching my nose and shovelling in a fork of pill-powder dust-food, then swiftly necking a mouthful of water to wash it down. It was commendable to provide patients with solid meals but I had real doubts about the nutritional benefit, not just the taste. That said, the highlight of my lonely Sunday afternoons was selecting meals for the upcoming week – with the realisation that having the ability to actually choose gave me a sense of autonomy.

When Saturday rolled around, I really didn't want to leave this retreat from reality. Knowing what lay ahead for me back in the hospital was almost enough to put me off. I was tempted to just say 'fuck it' and leave it all to fate. My only option, should I want to spend more time with my loved ones, was to return and face the music with dignity, focus on a future and ignore those niggling doubts that rustled around my feet like snakes in the grass.

Probation had ended. They'd recalled the prisoner. Mum escorted me back to the hospital in her trusty Nissan Micra. A quiet peace washed over me, the kind that comes from knowing what lies ahead. It was like walking down a track, through an ancient forest of dense green, no other humans around to make a sound. Retreading paths I'd already trodden, the squelchy footprints ahead half-full with cloudy rainwater, the ground soft and mushy underfoot.

My freshly-packed bag sat snug in the boot, along with two plastic carriers laden with home-cooked dishes. I'd store a couple in my fridge but there was also a freezer down the corridor. There was a microwave too; the nurses wouldn't mind heating me up something palatable once in a while. Another bag harboured the cartons of unopened nutrient drinks that I'd outright rejected. A little bit of rebellion went a long way towards keeping my sanity intact.

Ω

Angus & Kelly

Walking back to the bus, I picked up a scuffling sound from the rear of the diner. As I approached, the noise stopped, its instigator aware of my presence. I peered over a low wall and a small dog stared back at me, ears pricked, quivering slightly.

'Oh, hi there little guy.'

The dog scurried around the wall and ran at me full tilt, springing up and down at my legs, barking and yelping. Its muzzle twisted shape into what I could have sworn was a grin. Recognition hit me. 'Kelly? Is that you? What the hell are you doing here? It's cold, you'll freeze!' I knelt down to her level, ruffling her bristly coat.

Kelly was a black and tan mixed-breed, rescued by my parents from the streets of Leeds back in 1981. She'd been dead at least a year. It was a surprise to see her friendly face in this unfamiliar land. Scooping her up into my arms, we made our way back to the bus. Her tail wagged furiously. As the cowboy reached out to pet her, Kelly stretched forward from my protective cradle to lick his hand, glad to make his acquaintance.

'I see you found a friend,' he smiled, 'the more the merrier I say.' He patted her warmly, clearly won over by her sweet nature. He picked up his pipe. It was masterfully carved, its wooden bowl delicately whittled into a shapely body that narrowed into a slender mouthpiece. By far the most beautiful pipe I'd ever seen, clearly the work of an artisan. Without looking he drew a flame to it and took a slow hit. His lungs held for what seemed an inhumanly long time, until softly releasing a plume of sweet-smelling smoke that clouded the windscreen.

'I think it's high time we got ourselves some music on the go, what do you say about a bit of MacLise? Don't say "who?" – the man is a friend of mine, one of the old guard and a bonafide genius. Great times, great times…' he trailed off, shaking his head wistfully. 'Angus had the rhythm in him, like you.'

'I've never heard of him. What rhythm?'

The cowboy steered Dusty back to the highway. An unusual cacophony of hand-slapped percussive beats sounded off the walls like some chaotic ancestral ritual. A wailing violin began its quivering path to the higher reaches of the mix. The hypnotic repetition of the drums was punctuated by the sudden strum of an acoustic guitar.

Dusty's thirsty engine alternated between a purr and a growl, as his hulking metal chassis hauled us along the mountain roads. We must have climbed several hundred metres to this point. Turning in my seat, I saw the desert floor sharply drop away to my left. As we rounded a distinctly tight bend, fat drops of rain splitta-splatted against the windscreen. I caught a flash of my reflection in the glass, the face looked different to how I remembered. Kelly let out a whine and curled herself tighter at my feet. The clouds above swirled like squid ink in water, their forms unfolding and rolling out across the heavens with grand inevitability.

'Storms don't rage continually, nor is the wind forever boisterous; sometimes it blows fair and strong,' said the cowboy, reciting Somerset Maugham like a mantra.

'So where did you say we were going?'

'We've got a few things to take care of up in this valley.'

'Ah right, yeah. Cool.'

Of course. That made sense.

'Ride the King's highway, baby,' uttered the cowboy from under his breath, as the introductory bassline to The Doors' 'The End' drifted into the cabin.

Dusty's robotic wiper arms came into their own as the droplets grew fatter and faster, whipping the tiny rivers from one side to the next. The light of the sun was fading under the wet weight of the sky. Headlights illuminated a glossy road that snaked between two sections of dense pine forest, tailing a rocky stream back to its source.

We rumbled over a wooden bridge, then slowly down a steep hill to where the tree line thinned out abruptly by the shores of a glacial lake. A waving mass of bulrushes greeted us with their lazy dance. Hulks of rock rose dramatically on either side, their proud summits obscured by the heart of the storm. The water shimmered with ripples, oily and uninviting. A rough track hugged the water's edge all the way along to an imposing dam at the far end. I could just about make out the silhouette of a building next to it.

We drove in silence, no more music, no more drumming, no guitars. Just the staccato pounding of rain on steel above the steady whirr of Dusty's throbbing V8. The cowboy was focused and alert, his face etched with a determined grimace.

'We're gonna be parking up real soon kid,' he said, eyes darting from the road to the sky, 'and when we do, I need you to stick with me, ya hear? Don't go wandering off on your own in this place, it'll take your breath away.'

'It already has.'

'Ha! Good to see you've still got a sense of humour.'

'What? I wasn't joking.'

'Sure you weren't.'

Pulling up a short distance from the dam, the cowboy switched off the engine and stared seriously ahead. Kelly hopped onto the front seat, concerned, her furry ears tall and twitching. I stepped out and peered at the house in front of us, so much larger than it appeared from the other side. It was several stories high, more of a mansion than a simple dwelling. An ornate series of carvings nestled above the porch. The walls, windows, and doors were all black, making it almost invisible in the encroaching night.

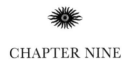

CHAPTER NINE

I See You

Of the six rooms on ward 23, I had already been a resident of two. On my return to hospital for the third and final round of chemo, I was placed in a different room. It was always a small thrill to get a change of scenery. Looking down there were no car parks in sight, only a few flat, grey hospital roofs below. In the near distance lay a smattering of trees and other greenery. These walls caught the afternoon sun, which gave it a lighter, airier feel. Apart from its view, room three was identical to room one, the only difference being its angular shape, which provided a more satisfying furniture arrangement.

Mum stayed for a couple of hours, drinking cups of tea and helping me settle in once more. After she'd hugged me goodbye with damp eyes, I sat on the bed watching Saturday sports shows on TV. Nothing much could hold my attention. I picked up a book and started to read, the sound of a golf tournament in sunnier climes hummed away in the background.

The door opened and a nurse I'd not met before came in. I guessed she must be agency – she wore a different uniform to the others, it was white with a blue trim, whereas all I'd seen before were varying shades of blue. The name badge read 'Helen'. She greeted me with a forced smile and a curt 'hello.' Helen's face matched her manner; sour and lumpy. As she took my blood pressure without even saying a word, I silently wondered where Luanne and Mary were. I was so used to their softness that in contrast Helen was spiky, less prone to smiling, and definitely not as up for a joke. I tolerated her more than I liked her,

Tasha had arranged to visit that evening, allowing me enough time to settle in and still have something to look forward to. Dinner was an unpleasant sandy slop of a chicken curry with starchy white rice. I'd yet to fill out my menu card, so I was served whatever spare dish was left on the trolley.

Trying not to watch the clock, I passed the time with a terrible talent contest, followed by a TV show in which the presenters themselves were the subject. I was catching up with the national news when 7.30 pm finally arrived. Tash burst in with a carrier bag full of goodies, slinging her brown leather handbag onto the easy chair and lighting me up with her smile. I swung my legs around to the side of the bed where she met me, planting a welcome kiss on my chapped lips. We spent a happy couple of hours trying to out-do each other at Scrabble, laughing at the innuendos we created, while scoffing on her fine selection of biscuits and crisps.

It wasn't quite 9 pm when Tash's dad rang, a punctual man who didn't appreciate being kept waiting. She left me with hope ringing in my ears, telling me to stay strong and to call her the next night. The family, minus her father for business reasons, were going on an impromptu holiday to Cornwall for a week the day after that. At five past nine, I was alone again with just my mind and the smell of Tash on my blue fleece jumper for company.

A steely determination lay underneath the brave face I'd fashioned. It was as if a part of myself I didn't know existed had taken control of my thoughts. I was still there holding the wheel, but the engine was powered by some other force. It lived inside me, propelling me forwards when I felt lost, picking me up from the toilet bowl when weak and flecked with vomit. I was not only becoming aware of its mounting presence but learning to place trust in it. This was unexplainable to anyone, even Tash. How I was mentally coping with the ordeal was never properly broached, except by the stranger who turned up unexpectedly later that week.

Mary was on shift. 'Jody, how are you pet? Would you mind a visit from the hospital chaplain? He comes round to see all our patients.'

'Do I have to? I'm not really the religious type.'

'No love, but give it a try, it might be useful, eh?'

'Ok, I don't see what harm it can do.'

She turned and nodded, and in shuffled a clean-shaven, smartly dressed middle-aged man wearing the white dog collar of a priest. He looked mildly uncomfortable. That made two of us.

'How are you doing, Jody?' he asked, adjusting his glasses.

'I'm alright, given the circumstances.'

There was something about this guy I didn't trust.

'I see. I'm, uh, here today to give you the opportunity to talk about how you are feeling. How you are dealing with the situation as your treatment progresses. Perhaps you are in need of some guidance?'

'Umm, not really, no.'

His expression faltered. 'So, have you thought, uh, about turning to the Lord for help? Turning to God?' he persevered.

'I haven't, no.'

'Would you consider letting God into your life at this time? I ask this of all the patients I see, we have a small team who come round to visit and lend an ear. When you are well enough, we also have a group that meets every week in the lounge next to the canteen on the second floor.'

'I appreciate the sentiment, Reverend. It's kind of you… but it's not for me.' I drew a breath. 'Right now, I feel like my strength to keep going with all this shit is coming from somewhere inside myself, not from any external force. Like, it's nothing to do with religion, it's coming from another place deep inside me. Quite incredible really. Do you know what I mean?'

His face wore surprise and confusion muddled with a dash of disappointment. Perhaps he was expecting someone in my condition to be more broken, with less hope and courage. Perhaps a desperate soul in need of a middleman such as himself to usher in the spiritual.

'Thanks for your time,' he mumbled, standing to leave. 'If there's anything more I can do for you please contact the chapel through one of the nurses.' He paused for a moment, then turned towards the door.

I felt strangely sorry for the guy.

'Well, at least you tried,' Mary said brightly, clearing the air. I couldn't tell if she was being sarcastic.

The third round hit me much earlier than the last. After a day of the new drugs I was flat on my back, my energy totally sapped, finding it increasingly difficult to eat. My sore mouth ached and had started to bleed in places. What food could stay down only sent my stomach gurgling, emerging an hour later from the other end. Never-ending sludge shakes and tablets of different shapes, coloured orange, white, and blue. I resumed my daily ritual of grinding them up and forcing them down.

This time my neutrophil count had been slow to climb. Doc Oc was taking no chances. I was only allowed out for a couple of days. I felt wiped out but happy to be home. As usual, Mum cooked up a couple of my favourite dinners. A visit from Tasha helped redress my mood. We lay on my single bed and she held me, planting kisses on my bald crown. She pressed a slim brown envelope into my hand as she left, telling me I wasn't to open it until I was back on the ward. Tash was always doing sweet things like that, even though I couldn't reciprocate. She lifted me. Despite the buoyancy in my heart from the short respite at home, I felt heavy as I climbed into our purple Renault Espace – quite some distance lay ahead on the road to a normal life.

Sat on my hospital bed with a cup of green tea, I carefully opened Tash's letter, a flutter in my heart. Out slid a card with a smiling psychedelic Lion, hand-drawn. The message read:

Stay brave, you're doing great! T xxx

Bruised and battered, I'd hung on until December. Two months into my treatment and I had faced everything that had been thrown at me. Copious chemicals had saturated my liver with toxins. I was a mere imitation of myself. Barely two months ago, that strong and confident young man had been on top of the world, flying high with love in his veins and dreams gathering in his big heart. He was happy. Now, this version of me was yellow-skinned and weak. Aches and pains sparked across my body, crackled around like tiny bolts of electricity. Mentally, I was coping but it was far from easy. Keeping myself positive had steadily become a gruelling task. It felt like a constant dance to both charm and fight my own flesh and blood.

Outside the hospital people were growing and changing, their lives unfolding each day as mine stagnated. Every now and again, I'd pass other haematology patients in the corridor. We'd share stories of our various personal ills, both exhausted yet directing what little hope we could towards one another. We were all in this together.

My treatment schedule often overlapped with a lovely lady staying in the room opposite mine, also from Bridgnorth. Jane had a chronic variant of lymphoma and was in her early forties with two young children, separated from her husband and three years of treatment behind her. She'd been in remission only to find the disease had come back for more. Her curly blonde hair was now a curly blonde wig, losing its ability to dazzle. Mum had met her at the local church and they'd often stop to chat on Saturdays in the middle of the bustling market.

We'd only spoken a handful of times but Jane was so positive and forward-looking. I admired her steely determination and easy laugh, and I made sure to check in whenever we crossed paths. Despite all she'd been through, Jane was well known by the nurses for her chirpy demeanour and fun-loving cheekiness. Once, while we were both bedridden, the cleaners wheeled us into the corridor so they could hoover and spray our rooms, fastidiously removing all the bacteria that might be lurking under the beds and around the furniture. We were both parked side-by-side for the ten minutes it took them to complete the clean. Time enough to talk frankly and openly about how we were coping, which drugs we were on, of the pains and nightmares we were going through. Having a friend who was also facing an uncertain future helped me apply a sense of objectivity in my outlook.

Doc Oc popped in with news that he was heading off to Cuba in a few days to speak at a haematology conference and would be enjoying a much-needed holiday afterwards with his wife. He declared himself happy with my progress.

After a particularly difficult night, I awoke with a dull ache down my right side. Attempting a deep breath, my lungs tightened and gasped for oxygen, sending a tickling cough lurching into my throat. I mentioned my discomfort to Luanne as she brought in breakfast.

She asked a few questions about my symptoms and told me she'd speak with Doc Oc about it when he came in. I was worried; my chest felt tighter and sleeping on my favoured right side had become uncomfortable.

A few hours later I felt a sharper pain. It began in the upper part of my chest and shot down towards my hips whenever I changed position. It set me off coughing again, like something was poking around inside my lungs, until I found it hard to breathe. I'd never experienced anything quite like it. The medication I'd been given for the pain did nothing.

A couple of hours later the doctor arrived. His flight was due to depart in the early evening, but he was still there at 1.30 pm, dashing around, arranging medications and somehow managing to monitor all his patients with a relaxed air of omnipresence.

Doc Oc listened closely as I described my symptoms and performed a thorough examination of my chest, rapping and tapping around my ribs and across my upper back, frowning with deep concentration. Deciding it was something to be investigated further, he asked me to reserve any mucus I coughed up. I should keep it in a small translucent pot for analysis. In the meantime, he prescribed a course of general antibiotics and made me promise to report any changes to the nurses, no matter how small, as soon as I felt them. Satisfied, he bid me a fond goodbye, asking me to keep well until he returned in seven days time. Until then I'd be under the care of another consultant, Dr. Murphy.

Throughout the following day, I expunged more and more phlegm from my burning lungs. My chest got tired. A steady flow of oxygen now passed through a plastic nasal tube to help ease my sleep. Dad stayed the night, sleeping next to me, solemn with concern. He fetched me iced water to soothe my mouth, helped slather coats of E45 over my drying arms and legs, and handed me tissues or a pot when my frequent splutterings woke us both up.

In the morning Mum arrived. Both of them were visibly worried, battling to stabilise their composure. The nurses monitored me closely, my condition growing progressively worse, the pain more frequent. They hurried me down to the radiography department for a chest X-ray.

That night the pain just kept coming, even the usually blunt Helen had softened towards me. The smallest movements now caused agonising, indescribable sensations around my torso. Several injections of strong painkillers had failed to do much more than sand-down the rough edges. The situation had quickly escalated. After a drum roll and a fanfare of precautionary warnings, out came the morphine. Housed in a small plastic box, a few milligrams were released at the press of a red button, roughly the size of a fingertip. It rushed through my body, numbing my nerves and clouding my brain.

On the fourth day, Dr. Murphy turned up, printout in hand, and sat down on the end of my bed. The blinds were still down from my afternoon nap. I felt Dad's support from the armchair next to me.

'Jody, we've had the results back from the latest phlegm analysis. What you've contracted is an aggressive form of Bacterial Pneumonia. I've been on the phone with Dr. O'Connor in Cuba and we've agreed that the best approach is to move you to the intensive care unit without delay,' he explained, pausing to gauge my reaction. 'This will enable us to monitor you more closely and react immediately to the slightest change in your condition.' He explained that their pneumonia specialist had recommended an intensive course of something called CPAP, which brought some unwilling grimaces from the nurses when my parents asked what that was.

The news hit like an anchor, weighing down our collective hopes. My mind started spinning. Intensive care has so many loaded connotations. It's where people die, isn't it? Where they take people on the very edge of life, the make or break level of the hospital game; you either come limping out the other side, nursing your wounds but still certifiably alive... or, you don't. Through a swirl of dizzying morphine, I let the realisation sink in that this was now an exceptionally critical situation.

I had become used to the reality of living with a disease, but adding serious complications made for a knife-edge scenario. The porters would be here in an hour to wheel me down to the unit as a private room was swiftly being prepared.

Outside the room and away from my ears, Dr. Murphy told Dad what he'd failed to mention in my presence: the situation was actually more complicated than they had first thought. Tests had revealed that my pneumonia had most likely been triggered by a significant MRSA infection. It couldn't have been much worse.

Luanne marched in. Her usual sunshine smile had turned sour, her cheeks the shade of a gently bruised peach.

'Jody, these two gentlemen are here to take you down to the ICU on your bed. I'll come with you and talk to the staff, we've secured a private room off the main ward,' she said, genuinely sad to be delivering the news.

'Am I okay to be there?' Dad interjected.

'Yes, I think that'll be fine, Steve.'

Opening both doors, Luanne stepped aside to allow a couple of burly porters into the room. The men set about freeing my bed in preparation for the move. Worries flooded in. I glanced over at Dad and caught a flicker of fear in his face.

'I'm with you,' he said stoically, gently gripping my arm, his usual positivity returning.

The scene was soft and dreamlike, enhanced, I'm sure, by the morphine. We rolled out down the bleached corridors. It was all happening in slow-motion. Was I not a little 'out of it', I'd have felt every squeak and buckle of the wheels as we swung yet another corner. The unmistakable hospital cocktail of shit and chemicals flooded my nose, daylight fading away as we reached what seemed like the farthest, quietest corner of the building. Heavy-set double doors marked the entrance. The ICU held a morbid gravitas.

Woozily, I listened as Luanne informed us about the CPAP treatment. It would start once I'd been set up in my room. Continuous Positive Airway Pressure is a direct and forceful method for opening up the lungs. As she explained the procedure, I felt what I can only describe as a cold wave of fear.

They would strap a tightly-fitting mask to my face, connecting me to a machine that would pump high levels of antibiotics mixed with oxygen directly down into my lungs. I wouldn't be able to breathe in or out on my own, and Luanne said I should try and allow the machine to ventilate me. It sounded like torture but what choice did I have… aside from having my throat cut open – commonly known as a tracheostomy – and put on a mechanical ventilator. It was a lot to wrap my head around, but it wasn't a tough decision.

The Shrewsbury ICU was a very dark place, both literally and metaphorically. The blinds were pulled low, blocking out the morning sun. There were about eight beds set out around a central nurses' station. Each patient had one foot in the grave. The few I managed to see had their eyes closed, motionless. One was ventilated, the colour drained from their skin. One had what I assumed to be family with them, praying, crying at their bedside. The stench of death hung heavy in the air. This could soon be me.

I was relieved as the porters wheeled me swiftly into my own private room, no doubt due to the high risk of further infection. Once again, my body was collapsing in on itself and needed a powerful intervention.

Dad stood outside the room, deep in conversation with Dr. Murphy who had come to support the procedure. The doctors were worried the pneumonia might cause acute pulmonary failure. They were prepared to use a ventilator if it came to it but would rather pursue the planned non-invasive technique first. CPAP increases lung capacity and the ability to absorb oxygen. It was also a delivery mechanism for the antibiotics that were needed to suppress the virus itself. No doubt I'd contracted pneumonia as a result of my seriously low immunity. For a patient in a neutropenic state, it was one of the most dangerous things that can happen. Becoming ill with next to no defences was one of my worst fears.

Within minutes, just as Luanne had said, two of the staff pushed in a large metal machine and began setting it up, pulling out tubes and wires and plugging things in. Dad was there the whole time, holding my hand. A dark-skinned man with a tidy beard approached my bed. He presented a full-face mask, asking if he could go ahead and strap it on. I nodded. It covered an area from my forehead to just above my chin. The mouthpiece forced my lips into a large 'O' shape – decidedly uncomfortable with the strange processed taste of hard plastic. The straps were pulled tight around the back of my head. Extremely tight. It hurt. My vision blurred. But once again I was ready to go along with it all. Whatever they needed to do to help me, I was fully onboard.

After checking their system, the man came over to brief me. I should try to relax and go with it. It would feel strange, he said, but it was very important that I gave it my best effort. They would do four sessions of five minutes each, with a one-minute break in-between. Through my steam-streaked mask, I turned to Dad. He gave me a brave smile and squeezed my hand.

'Ready?'

With a noise like a helicopter taking off from next door's garden, the CPAP machine whirred and clanked, and forcefully pumped an enormous torrent of air down the thick plastic tube and into my lungs. It briefly stunned me. The sound was intense. The mask was claustrophobic, I began to gag. It felt like I couldn't breathe yet I was taking in massive amounts of oxygen, a terrifying feeling that my brain struggled to compute. Thoughts of dying flashed before my eyes. Panic shot across my chest. I broke out in a cold sweat. After what felt like an eternity of this torture – but was probably just a couple of minutes – the violent airflow stopped.

'Well done, Jody,' the doctor said calmly. 'Three more to go.'

Fuck.

Breathing naturally again now felt weird. Dry as a desert, I could still taste the bitter antibiotic residue on the mouthpiece. The room was spinning.

'I don't... know if I... if I can do this...'

'We need you to do this, Jody, it's very important. Just another five minutes. You're doing really well. Ready?'

'Uh.... No...'

Back on it went. My chest expanded as the air rushed in. At this point, time condensed and I became unable to track the passing moments, as if in a whirl of hallucinatory excess. On with the third round, then the fourth. By this point I was almost entirely disconnected from my body. Then, thankfully, finally, it was over.

A woman leaned in, undid the straps and released me from the mask. She disconnected the merciless CPAP machine and packed it away. I lay there, propped up with pillows, drained and exhausted. Dad went to fetch some of my things from my other room upstairs, while the neat-bearded man set about attaching a series of monitoring devices. He gave me a gentle flow of oxygen through a thin plastic nasal tube and connected my IV line to a new drip stand. I was well and truly hooked up. Small LED lights flashed on the headboard above me and little bleeps sounded out a rhythm from the IV machine. I felt like a shell of a human, some sort of cyborg-hybrid being kept alive for strange experiments.

Had it worked? Was all that torture worth it? We simply had to wait and see. Throughout the night I would be monitored closely, dosed up on several different drugs. I began to lose my grip on reality. Everything was softly out of focus, just a blur of wires and white pillows. My breathing was shallow, but thanks to the self-administered morphine there was no real pain. A few taps of the little red button took care of that. I drifted into a thickly opiated sleep that would envelop me for the next few days. I felt safe knowing Dad was in the guest room next door.

My first night in the ICU and I was closer to death than I had ever been. It lingered in the darkened courtyard outside the window, separated from me only by a thin pane of smoked glass. It watched and waited.

In mythological terms, this was it; the big one. That fight the hero had been expecting for some time. With my adversaries so close, this was make or break, live or die. This was the moment to strike or be struck down. Could I follow this mythic narrative? Could I be the hero who outwits death?

Ω

Target Secured

'This is where you take the lead, kid. Ever used one of these?' The cowboy took an M-16 rifle from where it had been slung across his shoulder. 'Standard US Army issue, tough as shit. Guaranteed to stop 'em dead,' he said, thrusting it at me.

'Stop who dead?' I demanded. 'What's in there and why are we going in?'

'We aren't going in. You are. You know who they are, kid. I know who they are. These fuckers are not your friends, let me tell you straight. You see one of them, you shoot. Don't dare hesitate. That clear?' His southern drawl toughened.

'Very,' I replied. What the fuck had I gotten myself into?

'Don't be scared now, this is yours to lose.'

'Mine to what?'

'Don't think, just do. Ready?'

'Uh…. No…'

'Course you are,' he said, laying his hand on my shoulder. 'Listen here. You need to be on point for this one. It might get a little wild in there.'

The cowboy waved me onwards.

'Go steady and walk true. I'll be waiting right here. This next part is up to you.'

I stalked the house with a creeping fox-walk, cradling the cold metal with intent. It sat comfortably in my hands, as if I'd always had the use of it, as if it were a weaponised extension of my own body. The wind rushed through the valley; urging me on or pushing me towards a cliff-edge? I couldn't tell. Everything apart from Dusty was daubed in varying shades of black and grey, the sky a hulking slab of obsidian watched the scene unfold.

BOOM!

The doors blasted open. Out spewed a drove of formless creatures. They rushed towards me – suffocating, shrieking mist-beings. In an instant they were metres away.

'Fire, kid!' the cowboy shouted through the chaos.

Without thinking, I lifted the rifle, rested the stock against my cheek, scoped the swarming dark, and squeezed the trigger. I didn't feel a bullet leave and there was no kickback but I saw it rip into the creature and heard its death rattle. It had no face but I swore I caught a flash of anguish as my shot tore it from existence. Most lifeforms don't want to die and will fight to prevent their untimely demise. These things were no different.

My breath grew shallow and weak. I was scared and way out of my comfort zone but I somehow knew to keep going. The mission was clear; I had to get inside and take these fuckers right out of the game.

I spun around to look back at the cowboy. He was sat on Dusty's roof, smoking a cigarette.

'That was fucking crazy!' I shouted over.

He waved back at me, watching me walk on. Maybe the wind had taken my words.

Ok then. Let's do this. Lingering fears transformed into an adrenaline rush of chemical confidence. Driven to consume and destroy, these entities wanted nothing less. That would not happen, I decided. Over my dead body.

Blackened and burnt, the doors hung limply from their hinges. Inside, the house was quiet. An inviting orange glow emanated from a tall lamp at the far corner of the entrance hall. I hadn't seen it from the outside and felt relieved by the ability to contextualise my surroundings. The walls were stippled, ridged by some kind of irregular stucco. A mush of reddy-brown perhaps? Hard to tell. They seemed to be moving slightly, rising and falling like breath, with a sheen that implied they would be damp to the touch.

'Stay alert,' whispered a gruff male voice.

'Roger that,' I replied.

I made my way underneath an arched doorway that formed a short tunnel into the next room. Small sacs of fluid were trapped below the surface of the walls, bubbling like rising damp. My throat dried up. I coughed and hacked, trying to clear the irritation.

Something about the air in here – there wasn't enough of it. Like all the oxygen had been sucked clean out. I switched to breathing through my nose in slow sniffs, feeling the fine hairs inside my nostrils twitch.

There was no light up ahead, the shadows fading. I felt a cold sweat crawl up from my feet but urged myself head-first into the darkness, my trusty rifle cocked and ready.

'Are you still there?' I called out.

No reply.

A faint sound reached my eardrums – a hissing, bitter sizzle, coming from somewhere up ahead. Was that a faint crackle of radio static?

'Cowboy? Is that you?'

The hissing grew in volume as the temperature changed to a tropical humidity. I figured I must have left the tunnel but there was no way of telling. My lungs tightened. It was hard to draw a complete breath. The hissing contorted into a shriek and I realised the hidden predators were about to jump me. But from where? I couldn't see a thing. I hugged my rifle. More static. Piercing shrieks hit my ears and I started firing off rounds in a blind panic.

'Send a flare!' called a distant voice.

'Roger that!' came the reply.

'Give me a two and light it up.'

'Light in the hole, get down!'

A flash bleached the whole space. I threw myself to the ground. The beings retreated, blown back by the flare. Raising my head I could see maybe fifty of them cowering, trapped against a ledge on the far wall.

'Team one in position.'

'Team two moving in.'

The voices organised themselves.

I felt a heavy hand at my back. 'Target secured, fire at will,' said a voice from above.

A hail of machine-gun fire rattled overhead, fizzing across the space. Within seconds the hive had been eliminated.

'Team one, clear!'

'Team two, clear!'

'Secure the perimeter, prepare to move out,' said the gruff voice.

I rolled over and looked up. A towering officer dressed in pixelated camo, black combat vest, and fitted helmet stood over me. A khaki scarf covered his lower face but his eyes were kind.

'It's ok, kid, we've got your back,' he said gently. 'You're with us now.'

CHAPTER TEN

Morphine Dreams

That night in the ICU I had the first of my morphine dreams –
this is how I've come to refer to the days that I was in and out of
consciousness, struggling for life. Even when I was relatively 'with
it', a part of me was very much elsewhere, living out quests from
some other realm or parallel existence. It was an extremely intense
and visionary experience and is likely to stay with me for the rest
of my life.

That first dream awoke me. It was the catalyst in changing my
understanding of what it actually means to be alive. The doors of
perception swung open and a heightened awareness of the inherent
interconnectivity between my body and mind rushed in. I was lucid
dreaming before knowing what the term meant; an active participant
in the story that was playing out inside me. I was simultaneously
subject and object, I was at once God and a child of God.

You could say this was 'just a dream'. You could say it was solely the result of my bodily struggles that night, when the threshold between life and death was at its closest. But I lived it. While I would agree that the morphine embellished my visions, I truly felt it when we wiped out those dark entities. I could never write these dreams off as meaningless hallucinations or psychotherapeutic nightmares. I have no doubt whatsoever that those morphine-assisted, transcendental experiences directly impacted the recovery of my health, not to mention my chances of surviving the night.

The following morning Mum arrived. I foggily recall her looking at me, her frail first-born son, through the glass window in the ICU room door. Her eyes were puffy and tear-stained. She looked scared and tired in her regulation plastic apron. Mum describes the previous night as being 'the worst night of her life'. Dad had called to say they'd transferred me to intensive care. Afraid that I wouldn't make it through the night, she told him he must not leave my side, even for a second. That night Mum hardly had any sleep before waking in a cold sweat, feeling like she was having a heart attack, barely able to breathe. After sitting with my sister, Jemma, she felt able to call the out-of-hours doctor who assured them it was simply a panic attack. Mum was just about holding it together.

At the ward, an ICU nurse talked her through what had happened to me and how I was doing. But it was all just too much. Her son lay full of tubes and wires, teetering the edge of life, close to leaving this world. Mum burst into tears and had only just managed to compose herself when she appeared at my door.

It was difficult to see my parents so scared and upset. Instantly humbling. I felt compassion for their suffering and knew things must be very serious. I'd no idea of my appearance but could tell from Mum's face that it wasn't my strongest look. Part of me knew I was very close to death but I'd become rather adept at just being present to the endless treatments, accepting and trusting. From somewhere, I'm not really sure where, I had a reserve of strength to draw upon. I definitely shared my family's fears but the morphine had really taken the edge off, making life more manageable for me. I'm told that I was awake for no longer than an hour at a time before lapsing back into reverie once more.

That day I continued with the CPAP treatments. On went the mask and the straps were pulled tight. Somehow, I battled through it. Mum told me it was heart-wrenching to see me attached to that mask and be in the room when they activated the pump, forcing air into my lungs. She remembers seeing fear in my eyes, and as a mother wanted nothing more than to remove it. The nurses assured her it was helping me. Mum obsessively checked my oxygen saturation on the machine next to my bed, willing it to rise. The pattern of blips and bleeps steadily pounded out a monotonic rhythm of hope, like some sort of minimal techno in the dingy basement of an East-Berlin club.

I found myself in a large, open-plan classroom. It was similar to my school's common room where us sixth-formers spent most of our time. All my friends were there, sitting around on cushions and chairs. I was on my hospital bed in the middle. They were chatting and joking around. Everyone was smiling. There was an immense feeling of light and warmth, and I remember the entire scene being overlaid with hues of yellow and orange. They'd thrown a party, complete with cakes and drinks in cute cardboard cups. There was even a large banner strung high across one corner. In the dream, we stayed there all day. I felt so happy that they'd wanted to celebrate, that they'd all given up their time for me.

I opened my eyes blearily, not quite certain of the surroundings. What time was it? I had to get to the party before it was too late and I missed all the canapés and red wine. It was dreams like this that made the whole experience easier for me. I would awake from them feeling relaxed and happy, convinced they had been completely real experiences – little excursions away from the ward. Around this time, the differences between waking reality and the dynamic dream world became extremely blurry.

And then something very bizarre happened: I became utterly convinced that I could teleport myself. I discovered that whenever I pressed on a specific section of my upper chest, just below the sternum, it acted like an inter-dimensional launch button which instantly fired my dreaming consciousness out to wherever location I wished to be. It was fantastic fun. Unfortunately, it was not a popular thing to air in the intensive care unit.

The nurse who came to wash me and deal with my various bodily excretions just laughed at my newfound ability and dismissively told me it wasn't real. I saw her telling the other nurses through the window. They'd glance into my room, barely disguising their smirks. This all made me furious. Who were they to tell me what was real and what wasn't when they had no idea. How could they?

The only one who entertained my tales was a young Irish

doctor with floppy dark hair and a stubbly beard. He had soft eyes and must have been in his late twenties or early thirties. On his shifts he'd sit with me and ask about the teleportation: 'Where was I going? How did it work?' I told him how the other nurses had been laughing at me. He said they shouldn't be doing that and promised to have a word with them. I appreciated his sympathies and felt as if I had an ally. He was on my side and wanted to hear all about my adventures. I told him that I'd just spent a couple of hours hanging out at my girlfriend's house. We'd watched a film and been walking with her two black labs, then spent the afternoon lying in a big barn on a pile of dried hay making love. He smiled and told me it sounded wonderful.

The dreams I experienced were as real as being awake. In them, I thought, felt, and behaved as if I were completely conscious because I very much felt that I was. I travelled between these states in such a fluid and constant way that I quickly lost the ability to sense which was which. Perhaps my mind was protecting me from encroaching death as the borders between these worlds became almost translucent. Of course, the constant morphine top-ups I gave myself had played a role, but as the subjective experiencer, I can tell you that it felt more real than anything else I'd ever experienced. The memories of those journeys remain unusually clear and accessible to me, even now two decades years later I can pull up the scenes and recall how they made me feel.

I was sat up in bed, dozing, with Mum alongside me, reading.

Dad had returned home to look after my brother and sisters. Mum woke me gently, saying Tash was here and would I like to see her? Of course, I agreed, and suddenly her face appeared at the door's small square window. Tash had clearly been crying. Flushed and flustered, her bright blue eyes were streaked with dark eyeliner. Tear tracks ran down her cheeks but she was still smiling. I was overjoyed to see her. She came and sat down next to me, all wrapped up in plastic like a hospital sandwich. Mum left to get a cup of tea.

Tash kissed me and held my hand, gazing around at all the wires and lines and monitoring devices. Her eyes were full of worry, uncertainty. Seeing her brought me back into the waking world. I was still way out there in the borderlands of consciousness but somehow, she was able to keep me in the here and now, like an anchor between the worlds.

'Guess what Tash, this is so exciting… I can teleport!' I rambled. 'Now I can come and see you whenever I like, I just have to press this part of my chest…'

To her credit, she didn't bat an eyelid. 'That's great Jode, I'll look forward to it. I'm sure we'll have fun.' She smiled.

Tasha was great like that, instinctively knowing how to handle the most bizarre scenarios. We managed to have some semblance of a normal conversation, she told me everyone at school was thinking of me. Mr Phelps had mentioned me at morning registration and asked those present to hold me in their thoughts. Tash had brought in a card signed by all my friends, full of good wishes and loving energy. She gave me a kiss and left. Mum walked her out while Dad stayed with me, humouring my tales of romping through my wild dreams with his trademark stoicism and good humour.

Mum, however, worried I was losing it. I think she felt that allowing me to self-medicate with morphine was proving that little bit too tempting. Her views were compounded the following morning when she arrived to my wide-eyed tale of having teleported back home during the night and written off her red Nissan Micra on a quiet country lane.

'I'm so sorry Mum, it was an accident, there was nothing I could do.' I was sweating profusely.

She seemed strangely unaffected by the whole incident, a puzzled expression on her face. As far as I was concerned, it was clear as day. The fact that I was stuck in a bed in the ICU didn't seem to impede the flow of my logic.

'Jode, listen to me,' Mum said gently. 'The car is fine, you didn't write it off. It would be impossible since you've been here in the hospital lying in bed.'

'It's ok, you don't have to pretend. It definitely happened. I was there, I felt it. The front bumper was crushed.' I thought she was just trying to be nice. 'I'm sorry Mum, really I am, I know you loved that car.'

Mum welled up.

'You didn't though, Jode. You didn't write the car off, it's the drugs making you think that.'

'What drugs? What are you talking about?' It didn't make any sense. What I had done was not up for debate. I must have just got back before she arrived home, it was obvious.

'Why don't you phone Dad and check, he'll tell you,' I said, certain that he would corroborate the story. 'I promise I'll pay you back as soon as I can.' A terrible wave of guilt washed over me.

It took her another ten minutes to convince me that in fact, it wasn't true. She looked worn-out and defeated by my insistence in the truth of it all. Eventually, I grumblingly accepted she was right. Privately, I remained doubtful. Almost exactly a year later I actually did write-off her car off, in very similar circumstances. I knew I was right, time just hadn't caught up yet.

While I lived in this sleep-heavy, semi-conscious state, my parents would quietly speak to me. On one occasion when Mum was telling me their latest news, I slowly opened my eyes, as if waking to greet them, but stared straight ahead without acknowledging their presence. Oblivious to their frightened voices calling my name, I promptly fell back to sleep, right before their eyes. This disturbing moment took all of ten seconds and left them somewhat stunned. Mum was beside herself. The doctors came to console her and assured them that it was all perfectly normal and very probably due to the morphine. It was making my dreams so vivid, so realistic that they spilled over into waking life, animating my body as my awareness remained deep within the otherworld.

As my physical body fought with death, life surged within my dreams. I was in a hospital, different to the one I remembered. It was grand and shiny; each wall made of translucent glass. Everything felt futuristic and vibrant. Lying in bed, a nurse came running over and frantically told me that the band Feeder were coming to the hospital to kill me. With that, the three band members stormed into the lobby several floors below us, brandishing AK-47s, hell-bent on my destruction. The nurse helped me leave my room and I set out on a sequence of running around and hiding throughout the hospital labyrinth. It was getting serious. I had a strong feeling that if they caught me, I'd be dead. Really dead.

The fear cut deep, spurring me on and prolonging my life as various doctors and nurses aided my escape. It became clear that the musician-assassins were closing in and I knew something would have to happen. Somehow, I made it back to my room when Dad appeared. I told him, 'You have to help me' and he said he'd try and call his friend.

Meanwhile, the two of us made a break for it by squeezing through a small door that had materialised in the wall behind my bed. It led us outside the hospital building and around to the front. A large turreted wall stood opposite the main entrance. We scrambled up to find Jean Reno, star of the iconic Luc Besson film *Leon*, perched in one of the turrets with a sniper rifle. It turned out he was the friend that Dad had mentioned. We huddled down, trying to stay out of sight, keeping our eyes on the doors.

Before long, Feeder came running out of the building, angry and confused, thinking they must have lost me. Without hesitation, Jean Reno pulled the trigger three times – BANG! BANG! BANG! – killing each of them instantly. The sense of relief was incredible. Jean seemed pretty nonplussed about it all. He packed up his gear and made a sharp exit while Dad and I tearfully embraced and slowly made our way back to my room.

As I mentioned in the prologue, the language used to describe our relationship to disease – especially cancer – is often dominating.

My subconscious reflected this. Weapons and military imagery featured heavily, undoubtedly symbolic of the fight to stay alive. Those tripped-out dreams were windows into the internal, unseen processes that my body was undergoing.

While battle metaphors are a contentious issue in serious illness, I don't believe it's quite such a black and white, good or bad scenario. There has to be room for nuance. Space for people to make their own choices as to what feels right for them. My experience clarified why hard-fought conflicts are potent – and quite possibly innate – healing-metaphors. It was this very narrative that gave me the strength to work through the trauma and instill a sense of control as I surrendered to the primal survival instinct within.

Likewise, in the classic hero's journey, the protagonist must face a series of tests and challenges along the way, culminating in a final encounter. In my journey to the underworld, this manifested as a crack team of natural killer cells accompanying me on a mission to seek and destroy the pneumonia bacteria and MRSA virus, removing any trace of them from my body.

I've since come to understand that while the drugs had propelled me into a dream-state, my consciousness worked hard to process, translate and perhaps even influence my physical reality. On that first night in the ICU I could have decided enough was enough, welcomed the relief and silently floated away. It was then that my life truly hung in the balance. Instead, I found strength and focus. Becoming lucid in those morphine dreams positioned me on the front lines of the great battle that my body was constantly engaged in.

The ancient practice of fasting is undergoing a resurgence of interest from both the general public and the scientific community. This is due to a wider understanding of what happens when food is restricted for a period of time. After approximately twenty-four hours in a fasted state, the body begins the process of autophagy – literally meaning 'self-eating' – a natural regenerative process, a sort of deep cleaning that can help counteract the effects of ageing. Here's an excellent overview from the legendary Stephen Harrod Buhner's book, *The Transformational Power of Fasting*:

> *'Fasting allows the body to rest, to detoxify and to heal. During this time the body enters into the same kind of detoxification cycle that it usually enters during sleep. It uses its energy during a fast not for digesting food but for cleansing the body of accumulated toxins and healing any parts of it that are ill. As a fast progresses, the body consumes everything it can that is not essential to bodily functioning. This includes bacteria, viruses, fibroid tumours, waste products in the blood, any buildup around the joints, and stored fat. The result is that the body eliminates its toxin accumulation, just as during a fast the emotional and spiritual bodies eliminate theirs. And although fasting has been concerned with both spiritual and emotional healing, it has, as well, been recognised for millennia as one of the most powerful forms of healing for the body.'*

The latest studies have even found that fasting for seventy-two hours or more can result in a complete renewal of the immune system. I find this incredible. In 2018 the University of California ran a six-month study on both humans and mice receiving chemotherapy. Researchers noticed a significant improvement in their health, as white blood cells and other toxins in the body were flushed out during the course of the fast. They reported that the white blood cell count drops while fasting and increases once you re-feed.

The primary take-home, is that anyone concerned by the functioning of their immune system, either as a result of disease or ageing, can potentially utilise fasting to regenerate it. Why this knowledge isn't shouted from the rooftops, I do not know. Clearly, there is much to learn and integrate in the application of fasting as a treatment for disease.

Many indigenous traditions around the world – including Tibetan Buddhism, the Australian Aboriginals, and the Toltec in Mexico – hold the maxim 'life is a dream' as a foundation of their beliefs. According to such traditions, we are dreaming in the day as well as dreaming during the night. They believe we all possess a 'dreaming body'; an energetic field of awareness that ordinarily stays docked around our physical body. It can travel wherever it is projected; to the outer reaches of the universe, through endless dimensions, beyond time and space. This feels liberating and deeply inspiring. In their eyes, we aren't just a bag of blood and bones, 'walking meat sacks' as the American comedian Duncan Trussell often quips.

Taking this view, we can consciously access the magical, creative potential that we feel in vivid night dreams. We may begin to view life as a cosmic sequence, a flow of sorts. A dance between different dreams, accessed by simply shifting and adjusting our perception. If we can approach our lives with the perspective that each day is an unfolding dream, we ourselves become co-creators of a kaleidoscope of possibilities.

Ω

Innerspace

As an honorary SWAT team member I was kitted out with a spare walkie-talkie and a tactical combat vest, the pockets stuffed with grenades. They obviously thought I had some kind of explosives training because no explanation was forthcoming about how to use them. Then again, we were in the midst of a serious mission. Time was tight. The space had been cleared of death-mist-parasites, saving my life in the process. We'd moved on, working in tight formation, cleansing each and every room of the dark entities with ruthless precision.

The house began to morph as we swept through it, the rooms less flat-pack, less rectangular and more organic. It didn't look like any house I'd ever been in but there was something very familiar about it that I couldn't pin down. All very *Alice Through the Looking*

Glass, somewhere the Jabberwocky might hide out. If only I'd had a vorpal blade to snicker-snack my way through.

I thought about the cowboy, waiting outside. It wasn't the same without him but I felt safe with the SWAT team. They were organised and highly trained. Our enemies had raged and screeched but unlike us they had no tactics, no formation. Their wildness was their undoing.

'Clear to move!' came the shout from up ahead.

We entered what I took to be a kind of cathedral, fanning out into position. I looked up at the lattice of vaulted arches interwoven high above our heads, in awe of its magnificence. It felt reverential, holy, somewhere to pray. I was taken by the detailed architecture and the sense that it was somehow a living, breathing…

…and then the realisation hit, my vision sharpened, the depth of field expanding as if putting on a pair of glasses for the first time – I was dreaming. I snapped into life, into myself. What kind of reality was this? My awareness bulged at the truth of the situation – I had dreamed myself inside my own body. My lungs were under attack and here I was inside them.

Anger gripped me. This was my body. Mine. How dare they try and fucking infect me. I was ready to kill something, I had a life to protect. In the shadows above my head, the remaining mist-creatures lingered nervously.

'Up there!' I shouted, pointing to the rafters. 'Come on let's do this!'

From all sides of my lungs, our machine-guns rat-a-tat-tatted, their mechanisms crunched and whirred and blasted out the remedy to heal this sickness. Between rounds of steady gunfire and the shrieks of the dying, a welcome voice rang out with practised defiance, smoke-singed to a husky growl.

'Yeehaah! Go get 'em, kid!'

With the echo of his words still dancing about my ears, something shifted. I suddenly felt myself fall back. Ripped out of lucidity, the scene before me dissolved as I entered the void with nothing but a vague memory of the dream and the afterglow of adrenalin.

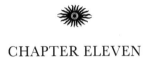

CHAPTER ELEVEN

Back to Reality

It was almost 3.30 pm in the afternoon. I'd been in the ICU for two full days. Tasha sat on my bed, gazing through the window into the courtyard opposite, lost in thought. A noise startled her and she turned to look at me. My eyeballs flickered underneath their lids, a soft moan escaped my throat and I rose back into the world as I'd left it, dazed and not quite sure of my surroundings.

I took a while to adjust to the freshness of the light. Peering at Tash, I slowly realised who she was and felt a spark of happiness. My body was still warm and fuzzy from the morphine. Over the course of the preceding day – and without my knowledge – the nurses had removed the pump and begun weening me off with lower and lower injected doses.

'Hello you.'

'Hey gorgeous,' I croaked.

'How are you feeling? You've been dreaming for days. The last time I visited you were pretty out of it.'

'Really? Shit, I can't remember much after those hardcore mask-drugs. I feel a bit better though, breathing doesn't hurt as much.'

'There's definitely a bit more colour in your cheeks,' she said, leaning over to kiss me lightly.

'I've had the *craziest* dreams, Tash, you wouldn't believe them if I told you.' I ran my forefinger over my lips, feeling the ridges of chapped skin. 'Is there any water around, my mouth is really dry.'

I drank gratefully in several thirsty gulps. Tasha looked at me, glowing with love. The strain of her experience was etched across her face. I saw all she'd been through to support me and all that she'd sacrificed to be at my side. No matter if her own day had been a hot mess, her consistently encouraging voice was always at the end of the line. Her cheerful nature was guaranteed to lift me.

We kissed again, longer and with tenderness. Her blue eyes welled up and began to drip onto her clean white shirt. Immediately, I realised part of me had made it through simply to receive that kiss. I still couldn't believe she was actually sticking through this journey with me, this beautiful shining girl. Where had she come from? What had I done to deserve her? She made me feel bolder, stronger, calmer. She was my anaesthetic, and she took my pain away.

'I love you,' I blurted.

'I love you too.'

Through teary declarations, giggles emerged. Her laugh was contagious, it brought hope back to the room. The air had cleared.

There was a knock on the door and in came the young Irish

doctor. He was the only one who'd gone along with my fantastical stories and my newly-discovered ability to teleport. He smiled kindly at us, genuinely pleased.

'So you're back in the land of the living then, eh Jody? You've had a good old rest there.'

I smiled weakly.

'You'll be pleased to know the latest lab tests have come back, and your pneumonia's almost been kicked out. We've got to keep a close watch on your breathing and keep you on a course of high-level antibiotics, but I think with Dr. O'Connor's approval we should be able to let you go back up to your room on the ward in another day or two. I bet you can't wait to get out of this place, eh?'

'That'd be really good.' I grinned. Tash looked at me proudly, smiling her sad-eyed smile. I couldn't tell if she was about to start crying again.

'Well that's all I wanted to say right now, you've had a tough time of it this last week and you've got a lot of rest and recovery still to do. I'll come back and explain more about what's going to happen when your parents are next here, but for now, I'll leave you two alone.' He winked at Tash, who blushed a pretty crimson and wiped the wet patches from her eyes with the back of her sleeve. With that, he left, a clipboard tucked neatly under his arm and a spring in his step.

After several consecutive days of existing in a liminal space between waking and dreaming, I noticed that I was more 'here' than 'there.'

More awake than in-between. I could think clearly and rationally again, coherently answering questions, and had started to feel more connected with my waking self. Despite my growing sharpness of mind, I refused to deny the seemingly illogical teleportation episode, reserving several scornful looks for the nurses. A degree of laughter was still detectable in their eyes and it cut me.

Coming round was such a rich cocktail of emotion and sensation. On one hand, I was happy that the doctors had shifted out of panic mode. I'd somehow come through a meeting with death and my battered body now showed the first signs of recovery. Everyone was relieved. Mum and Dad were understandably still shaken. I guessed they didn't want to get too optimistic too soon, perhaps trying to protect themselves should things take a turn for the worse.

That week left me with so many questions and so much to process. I had a vague sense of significance about what had taken place. Forcing my understanding of it would only diminish it's presence.

Doc Oc had been away in Cuba throughout the week, kept informed about my condition by phone. On his return, he landed at Birmingham Airport, sweeping into the ICU the next morning, joking that I must have deliberately timed contracting pneumonia to coincide with his first holiday in a year, just to stress him out. Under all that bluster, it was evident he was very relieved I was still alive. To have one of his youngest patients die whilst he was thousands of miles away would have surely weighed heavy.

He told my parents that they were almost on top of the pneumonia virus but the MRSA was still causing problems. My cancer treatment couldn't resume until I was free of both infections and well-rested. Dr. Murphy described how the morphine had knocked me out cold, that I'd hardly been awake for more than an hour at a time. It was better I was resting and free of pain, giving my body a way to recuperate while the other drugs did their work.

Up until this point, the nurses had assisted me in all of my basic hygiene needs. Several bed baths a day helped me feel less disgusting. After another day of tests the notorious commode had been retired and I was able to visit the toilet unaided, my dignity somewhat restored. I had to lean on Mum to get there and she waited outside until I was done, but by God was that a personal victory. I hated being lifted onto that portable poo-station, sitting there crapping and wincing, zoning out as a nurse stood by. If only I could have seen myself at that point. I hadn't seen my reflection in a week and really wasn't looking forward to the face that awaited me.

The next morning, they decided I was well enough to leave the ICU. My bed was detached from all the wires, wheeled back up to the ward by the hospital porters. Glancing around at those less fortunate, the frail and half-dead, I counted my blessings, feeling beyond lucky to get out alive. I'd won. But what exactly? No idea, but it was decidedly bittersweet. I tried to focus on the sweetness.

Back in my room, the friendly porters parked me up and I flicked on the TV, desperate for some mindless distraction. Mum popped down to the cafe to grab a coffee. Before Richard Madeley could launch into his 10 am tirade about something completely frivolous, Luanne knocked on the door. She came in and sat down next to my bed.

'Hey, we missed you Jody, how are you feeling? We've all been so worried about you up here, the ICU nurses were keeping us updated.'

She looked at me sweetly but with real concern in her eyes and I felt yet another level of care and support. Another layer of kindness to wrap around myself. As Luanne reattached my monitoring devices and plumped my pillows, she didn't seem like my nurse in that moment, more like a friend. Her brightness brought me out of my head and I even managed to crack a couple of self-deprecating jokes. Progress.

'Alright soldier?' said Mary cheerily, heading over to perch on my bed. 'You gave us quite a scare,' she said, taking my hand, looking me in the eye with a warmth that simply said *I'm glad you made it.*

'I've made a little something for you, I make them for all the patients, keeps me out of trouble with the husband, you know.' She winked.

It was a knitted red and green striped cover for the plastic bag of drugs that swung from my ever-present IV stand. It was as cute as it was kitsch, yet utterly charming.

'It's getting close to Christmas and this place can always do with a little dose of festive spirit.'

'Ah thanks Mary, that's really sweet of you.'

She batted away my gratitude with more kindness. 'Would you like a shortbread? I made them on Sunday for Uncle Len's birthday and had a whole box left over.'

'They're really good!' Luanne called over her shoulder as she left the room.

I smiled. I was glad I'd made it too. I felt fractured, yet the dramatic inner journeys I had undergone had somehow empowered me. The dreams showed me a new level of self-belief was possible. An awareness blossomed that the foundations for healing lay within myself, that my mind and body could work together in a mysteriously complex way. I'd always been fascinated by dreams and the messages that they present. My raucous morphine dreams had expanded my sense of self. I felt more connected to life. I was learning how to listen to this other language, one of symbols and gut feelings – that sense of inner-knowing and guidance that we're all able to tune into if we just take a moment to try.

I was raised with a keen love for the outdoors. Our family walks took us all over the British Isles, a prime and cherished feature of my childhood. Despite plenty of moaning and grumbling about everything from the length of the journey up to Northumberland, to the quality of Dad's hastily-thawed fish-paste sandwiches, those adventures are stored firmly in my heart.

As a teenager, I played hockey for Bridgnorth's local team, marauding up the pitch from my position as a right-back. You had to be fast, agile and quick-witted to stay on top. Since the age of eleven I had slowly been developing into a skilled drummer, a passion which eventually crowded out my other hobbies by the time I was sixteen. The most physical of instruments, drumming had helped me develop a strong upper body, giving me the confidence that I needed. I played in a band with my friends, enjoying the spike in popularity almost as much as the music. But after several weeks in hospital, my poor intestines shitting themselves inside out, the intermittent vomiting, and the toxic chemo, my physique no longer reflected any of that. I felt far from attractive. Far from a man. My overriding concern was that Tasha would think I was an ugly, stinking mess and want nothing more to do with me. In fact, that was the main cause of my fluctuating moods, rather than the illness itself.

On one occasion, Tash visited with a few items she'd been asked to pass on. I'd been sent several cards and letters of well-wishing support which brightened up my world.

The former head of special needs at my school, Jon Smith, is a very sweet man. Never short of a smile or a quip, Mr Smith bimbled about the place in his own cheerful way, never seeming to take anything too seriously. All the kids loved him. An accomplished blues guitarist, he'd frequently join in our after-school band practices, and in the corridors between lessons we'd often chat about music, sharing newly-discovered artists. He could enthuse about the Johns Mayall and McLaughlin for hours.

Jon had written me a lovely letter of encouragement. In the envelope was a cassette, a mixtape he'd made containing a hand-picked selection of his favourite tracks. I was touched that he'd taken the time to do something so thoughtful. I listened to that tape a few times a week and still have it to this day. It's the primary reason I've retained a peculiar fondness for early Dave Matthews Band records.

While I was in the ICU, Tash had dropped off a card signed by all my friends at school. Now, days later I actually had the energy to read it. Their messages were heartfelt, with some welcome silliness from the usual suspects.

Get well soon Jody, we miss you – Lucy x
Stop skipping school Mr Drummer! – Rishi

I pictured them all, beaming their love towards me. Another simple but effective action. Knowing that people out there were thinking of me was a reminder I was not alone in all of this. It wasn't just me and my family battling against the Big C. I had backup, I had a support team.

The wave of positivity being sent my way also included traditional religion. Mum has been a regular Church of England patron for most of her adult life. Far from your average tow-the-line Christian, Mum maintains that the idea of a benevolent God gives her solace. It brings the connection to a higher power that I think most humans seek, consciously or otherwise. Singing a stirring hymn gives her joy and her churchgoing fulfils a need for community. I know she prayed for me at home and at the local church where the vicar would ask his parishioners to hold me in their thoughts.

My grandparents also have a Church of England background and would say their prayers for me every Sunday at their service in Hinckley, Leicestershire. Mum's cousin Peter, before he retired, used to be a minister. He's one of those guys in the extended family you might bump into at funerals. The first time we met was at the reception following my Grandma's cremation, several years later. A warm man with dancing brown eyes, he introduced himself, enquired about how I was doing, and told me how he'd regularly ask his congregation to pray for my health and healing. My heart near burst with love and gratitude for this man. What kindness – we were strangers really but connected through our bloodline.

Having all this coming my way felt humbling. Although I don't believe in the concepts of Heaven and Hell, or that to die well I must be saved from sin, there is something undeniably powerful about the united effort to direct love. I have no doubt that I received their prayers and that they impacted my state of wellbeing, perhaps even the ultimate outcome of my treatment. Entirely unprovable of course, and the sceptics would rip such a theory to pieces, but the power of prayer is a satisfyingly mysterious yet well-documented phenomenon. It takes us outside the bounds of accepted scientific reality – where something only exists if it can be measured – and is therefore easily dismissable by those who follow a strictly logical doctrine.

If you listen closely to your heart on this matter, you might just hear the echoes of an inner understanding that prayer, or the act of focused ritual intent, has power far beyond what we've been led to believe. After all, science, in the form of quantum theory, has already shown that everything in the universe is energy. It doesn't take too much of a leap to see prayer as a form of sending energy.

You could clarify this as: 'directing conscious intent with a clear and focused mind.' This is the key. Working in this way, especially when combined with breathwork, can be extremely effective – you send out a clear energetic message. Life – or the powers-that-be – will hear, listen, and respond. How that response comes back is an unknown. This is where the trust comes in.

This technique of holding an intent lies at the root of all ritual and ceremony, practices inherent within esoteric spirituality and all traditional religions. You don't have to belong to a formalised group to access it. I've found the practical and mindful aspects to this process immensely beneficial in our overtly stimulating world. We have forgotten – some would say *trained to forget* – our arcane roots. Anyone and everyone can tune into the multi-dimensional, timeless web of life and tap the wellspring of potential miracles.

A week had passed since I'd left the ICU. Still wooly, all I could tell was that I was deeply tired. Not tired in the way you are when you get home from work, not even in the way you feel after an hour lifting weights, but a whole other kind of tired. The sort that is barely possible to imagine. My entire being ached, as if I'd been forced to run marathons while I slept each night. Every hollow bone and taut sinew, every snapping nerve and silently pulsing synapse told my body's sorry story. Yet from this place, over time, somehow I regained my strength.

It was now mid-December, the time of the year when our society revolves around the re-appropriated pagan festival slash capitalist wet-dream called Christmas. That said, I do love a celebration.

As my recovery progressed, Doc Oc sent me for a series of radiotherapy sessions, aiming to complete this last stage of his treatment plan before the Christmas break. Too weak to walk, a hospital porter would wheel me down to the second floor, to a suite of shadowy rooms in what felt like a subterranean department.

Before the last one of these sessions, my good friend Ben came to visit. That kind-hearted kid even wheeled me down there in my wheelchair – thanks mate. He appeared nonchalant with the whole situation, trying not to show that this was actually a really bizarre thing for two teenage lads to be doing. I could tell the gritty reality had shocked him a little.

Once inside, I undressed and glanced out through the small glass window. Ben was sat down, flicking through a well-thumbed copy of *People's Friend*. The technician got me to stand in my underpants in front of a flashing, beeping machine while he retreated to the safety of an adjoining control booth, no doubt reinforced by thick layers of protective material. I was then asked to take a deep breath and hold for ten seconds as a barrage of frequencies blasted my pale, wilting skin.

These radio waves glide powerfully and effortlessly into the very cells that our organs are made of. Their job is to permanently damage the DNA of the cancerous cells. This is all well and good, but as with chemotherapy, it can't help but affect the healthy cells too, especially those nearest the treated area. I didn't want to think about the long term damage. I still don't. It's not a pleasant experience, but again, I had little choice but to trust the doctor and his procedures. I had to trust my body's ability to heal, repair, and rebuild itself further down the line, should I come out the other side.

Radiotherapy made me extremely tired. The chemo was exhausting, but this was another level. I wanted to do nothing but rest in bed. A few days later and my energy levels had all but flatlined. Underneath all this came a surprise: I noticed I was feeling happy. A wave of positivity had spread through me and I felt buoyant for the first time in months. The simple fact that I had not yet died gave me a renewed sense of hope.

This was compounded further by news delivered by a very cheerful Doc Oc one grey and frosty morning. He bounced into my room with a grin on his face. This was nothing new but there was a slight spring in his step so we all sensed something was about to be revealed.

'Well, Jody, I have some good news,' he said, trying not to look too pleased. 'Your leukaemia is in remission. I've just got the latest test results back and we can safely say that this is the case. There appears to be no trace of the leukaemia cells in your blood or bone marrow. Now...'

Mum, Dad, and I looked at each other and broke out in smiles of pure relief. I saw Mum's face visibly release some of the tension she'd been holding onto since the day of my diagnosis. The lines on her forehead withdrew. Her eyes softened as Dad squeezed her hand.

'At this point, I must state that this doesn't mean you are cured,' he added. He paused, allowing us to take this in. 'What it does mean is that the treatment so far has succeeded in stopping your cells mutating and has removed the leukaemia cells from your body. The levels of these cells are now all but invisible. However, we don't usually advise our patients to stop here. You have made very good progress, but if we want to go for the best possible chance at a long-term cure we would be looking at a bone marrow transplant.'

We were silent. It sounded huge. We'd all known this option was a possibility but it hadn't prepared us for the reality of it actually happening. Part of me had been secretly hoping that it wouldn't be necessary. It scared the hell out of me.

Doc Oc continued, 'We don't have the facilities for that here, so you'd need to go over to Birmingham, to the Queen Elizabeth Hospital for that. A very good friend of mine leads the department there – Dr. Prem Mahendra. She's one of the top haematologists in the country so you'd be in very good hands. Of course, it's completely your decision but I would really urge you to explore this option to prevent the leukaemia returning later on down the line.'

We exchanged weighted glances. He didn't need to carry on, I got it. Mum and Dad immediately understood too. If Doc Oc says I should do it then it's happening. I had trusted this man with my life one-hundred percent and he'd helped get me this far. If a bone marrow transplant was the best chance towards freedom from this disease then why not take it? I knew there were risks but I could feel in my heart that this was the next step, the way to close-in on the goal of being cancer-free. I signed some forms, Doc Oc made some calls and that was that. I was going to Birmingham in the New Year.

Sitting in my hospital room on December 23rd, just before my parents arrived to take me home, a thought struck me: *what if this was to be my last Christmas?*

No, don't be stupid, I'm getting better, Doc Oc told us so. I'm in remission.

But you aren't cured… nothing is certain.

That's true, but there's a whole other stage of this treatment on the horizon, I just need to rest and then I'll be ready for it.

Hah, you aren't out of the woods yet kid!

Christmas. That strange and emotional time of year where many folks get together to remember their love for one another. On the other hand, it can also perpetuate feelings of loneliness and disconnection. The Christian church would have you believe that it's about remembering the birth of Jesus Christ, Son of God, who lived a couple of thousand years ago. Aside from the token televised carol services and a few school nativity plays, I'd wager that not so many of us are actually that bothered about celebrating his birthday.

In the modern age, the Christmas period has mutated into an international, cross-cultural spend-a-thon. It's extremely hard to avoid the sheer hypnotism of it. All that buying generates more revenue for retail businesses than at any other time of the year.

It can be a time of deep remembrance and forgiveness, yet every year there are people freezing at home without money to pay for heating, or out on the streets going without proper shelter, food or sleep, while inside in the warmth others luxuriate in the trappings of a financially unsound spending spree, brains poached in excessive quantities of alcohol. Everyone seems to indulge in this cultural hypnotism, hangover be damned. Truth be told, it's a festival no-one really knows why they're involved in, other than perhaps the fact that the collective momentum around it appears unstoppable.

For me, Christmas has always been about loved ones. In my family, we are blessed. Lucky enough to have developed our own cute traditions over the years: the ritual displaying of papier-mâché nativity figurines, handcrafted by me and my sister when we were kids; the ceremonial dressing of the tree with eccentric decorations hidden amidst the candy canes. We'd wake to a full stocking outside the bedroom door, larger gifts mysteriously arrived in the porch early on Christmas morning, allegedly delivered by the big man himself. We didn't go overboard on the gifts like some families, with four kids my parents couldn't afford to, but nevertheless it was an indulgent time. A time of too much TV, good food, and too many

Cadbury's Roses. It was also a time of much hilarity and warmth, and we all really looked forward to it.

Christmas in 1999 was, as you might imagine, just plain weird. A dichotomy of bittersweet pleasures. What had always been a fun and light-hearted occasion in former years was now stained with an uncertain question: would Jody live to see another one? We could all feel it. It coloured every single moment. But being British we soldiered on regardless of the enormous elephant in the room. We didn't address the subject and perhaps that was a better way to deal with it. We all wanted to have as normal a family Christmas as possible given the strain of the last few months. Mum busied herself cooking up all sorts of meals, puddings, dips, and cakes. Despite the huge stresses she'd been under, she refused to let it bring her down, somehow channelling her energies into creating a homely and cosy environment in which we could all simply be together. To gift us the perfect Christmas must have been a tremendous pressure.

For those brief times when the family were together, in spite of our pain, it felt like nothing could stop us. The experience had strengthened our bond. We were stronger because we had each other. It cemented a deep feeling of trust. As I recall, we didn't have a great deal of outside help. Friends and colleagues supported at an unsure distance. Aunties, uncles and grandparents would phone to check up, occasionally visit me and look after the other kids. In no way is that a complaint or a judgement, it is simply a summation of the situation from my admittedly hazy perspective. Only the immediate family knew the true impact of what we were going through. But that didn't matter, we were strong enough to weather this storm.

On Christmas Eve, Tash paid me a flying visit. Being stuck in hospital I hadn't got anything for her in return. I felt embarrassment flush my face as she buzzed in and out of the house in a flurry of blonde streaks and ripped blue jeans. Seeing her energised me. It always did. We'd planned to spend a little more time together on Boxing Day afternoon. I was scheduled back into hospital on the 27th and wanted to see her properly before then.

As Christmas Day rolled around, spirits were on the rise, from our traditional breakfast fry-up to the very last sips of bedtime brandy. We ate, they drank, and all of us were surprisingly merry. Presents were shared and trashy TV-specials were dutifully observed. Those simple things you take for granted each day become so much more important when life hangs in the balance. The luxury of sitting around the dinner table together with my family, tucking into, or in my case gingerly picking at, a feast of turkey with all the trimmings brought its own degree of healing. For a family shaken to the core, this celebration was needed.

Making the journey along the twisting A349 between Bridgnorth and Shrewsbury for the last time in 1999 was a little less depressing, recharged as I was by the indomitable force of my family's love. The year's end felt more than a little significant and I couldn't wait for it to arrive. I was ready to move forwards. My focus had to be on resting, building my strength, and mentally preparing myself for the challenge of the bone marrow transplant. In truth, I'd done incredibly well to make it this far. Now I had a chance of making it all the way, of really beating this thing. It all hinged on finding a suitable donor match.

> **From:** Tash
> **Sent:** 11:03 am
> In Somerfields stocking up on goodies!
> See you around 7:30 gorgeous xxx

December 31st, 1999 remains one of my most memorable New Year's ever. Mum, Dad and the siblings came to visit, still buzzing from our time together, before heading out for a celebratory dinner in Shrewsbury. I was looking forward to a special night of my own. A few weeks prior Tash had gently asked if I'd like to spend New Year's Eve with her. At first, I'd got confused and then realised what she was suggesting. She wanted to come and spend the night with me in hospital, to make this transition into the year 2000 one of our own. My heart fluttered. God, how I loved her. Then guilt took over. I didn't want her to feel duty-bound to come all the way over here, spend her evening sat on a hospital bed with her skinny bald boyfriend when she could be out with friends, enjoying the year's biggest party. I didn't want anything out of pity. She insisted that what she wanted most of all was to wake up with me on New Year's Day. Nothing else would do.

What a gift; a sincerely beautiful offering. Once again I saw the purity of her heart and understood a little more about how it filled me up in such moments. She knew what it would mean to me and had planned it perfectly, even bringing a VHS player. There'd be films, games and snacks, and plenty of snuggling up. Simple. We ran the plan past Emma who smiled knowingly and said of course it'd be okay, how lovely an idea it was. Luanne kept shooting me hilariously unsubtle winks. They thought she was as amazing as I did.

Just after midnight on the first morning of the year 2000, after a wonderful night of love and laughs, Tasha asked if I felt up to going outside. I probably wasn't, but it felt like a rare moment in time. She layered me up with blankets and helped me into the wheelchair. She put my new bobble hat on, a Christmas gift, and pulled it firmly over my ears. I'd developed quite the collection of knitted beanies by this point.

'Don't stay out there too long,' Luanne said motheringly, as we slowly made our way along ward 23 to the lifts that led to the ground floor.

Out we went through the front doors, turning left towards the nearest bench. The night sky was oiled black and spotted with stars. Tash lit a cigarette, took a drag and slowly exhaled. We stayed in the silence for a minute. All my senses were alive. Everything became extremely vivid.

Looking at the stars never fails to enchant me. Those little specks of flickering light burning millions of miles away. The realisation that you are but a tiny human on a tiny planet is impossible to ignore. On a universal scale we are but particles of dust.

I thought about the storm I'd been swept up in the past few months, all that blood, shit, and tears. October felt like an eternity away. At that moment, an ambulance screeched to a halt right outside the main doors. We looked on as the paramedics rushed to get the patient transferred to a trolley. It seemed pretty serious. They swept the patient out of the van and into the hospital in a whir of bodies, luminous jackets, and machinery. As the hustle and bustle died down, I was reminded just how lucky I was. Here at the breaking of the year's first day, this guardian angel beside me, the heavens dancing above. Looking up at the sky I felt a bright future calling me through the distant pinpricks of shimmering light.

Ω

The Dark Moon

Dusty woke with a stuttering purr as the cowboy hit the ignition. It was still dark but the sky had softened towards a new morning. The clouds, purple-grey and plump like hotel pillows, had begun drifting beyond the towering dam wall in a north-westerly direction. It was time to leave.

'Get us home safe now,' the cowboy said, letting out a deep sigh.

It had been a long night and he was ready to rest his aching bones. He thought of the boy, in there fighting with all his heart.

They trundled along the track that led away from the house, feeling the jolt from every rut and stone. Dusty's luminous orange curtains shimmied this way and that, their edges flicking up. The cowboy gripped the wheel, his eyes fixed gently on the road, lips curled up in a half-smile.

Re-tracing the route up, they wound back down the mountain

road, through boulder-strewn glades of arrow-straight pine and eucalyptus. Beyond the trees, they rounded bend after bend, past dozens of thorny shrubs and wizened cacti, dotted across the hillside like freckles.

Descending further, the vast plains of the desert unspooled, rolling out as far as the eye could see in a humbling display of grandeur. The cowboy allowed himself a full-on grin. He'd always loved the silent drama of this particular view. Dusty slowed to a crawl then stopped, engine idling. The cowboy drank it all in. The air was crisp and thin. He inhaled deeply, as if taking his first real breath for weeks, and surveyed the landscape laid bare before him.

Gazing across the plains, it was just possible to make out a small cedar-framed cabin, hiding in the sprawling vastness of the desert scrub. A mossy slate roof, partially obscured by trees, was given up by a wispy plume of wood-smoke rising from the chimney.

Inside, a plump old woman stood by the burner and slowly stirred a deep copper pot, filled half-way with a bubbling liquid. She hummed a simple looping melody. The lines about her face spoke of stories she no longer told – stories of another time and another place. Her stiff grey hair held the musk of earth.

Lost in her song, she busied about the kitchen, selecting and measuring different herbs and roots which she added to the pot with practised aplomb, whispering words of thanks to each ingredient under her breath in an extended incantation. Thus began her Dark Moon ritual. Blessing the brew she stepped back, put the lid on, and turned to the window. The sun was setting and the clouds were gathering in. Deep orange and yellow hues shone across the assortment of skulls, feathers, and small stones that lay gathered in piles on the ledge.

Dusk was poised to unveil itself as the precursor to a long night without stars. As if to define this threshold had been passed, the unmistakably mournful howls of a wolf pack rang out across the desert floor in chiming unison, singing the timeless songs of their ancestors.

CHAPTER TWELVE

Transplant

As the new millennium began in earnest, I remained at Shrewsbury Hospital. Before they could officially sign me over to the care of the Queen Elizabeth in Birmingham, I had a couple more spinal injections to endure. Luanne had told me I could expect to be allowed home in another couple of weeks.

In the first week of January under a cold grey sky, my three siblings came in for bone marrow testing. It was standard procedure to test the immediate family before looking anywhere else. They each had to undergo the delights of a lumbar puncture. I assured them it wasn't that bad. The samples would then be sent off to a specialist lab.

My parents brought Jemma, Jessie, and Josh up to the third floor to say hello briefly before their appointments. Seeing their brave, expectant faces sat around my bed warmed my heart. I felt grateful to my parents for creating this family. They were all here for me, determined to be the one who could help. Mum stayed with me while Dad took them to get their tests done.

Josh, only six at the time, didn't have much of a clue about what was going on, other than it was pretty serious. He'd not been into a hospital since birth, and I think the whole procedure freaked him out somewhat:

'One of my strongest memories was of getting the blood test. I remember really disliking the sensation, it was as if I could feel the blood throughout my whole body being sucked towards this tiny needle-sized hole in my arm. As soon as it was over, Dad took me out of the room where I think I fainted and proceeded to throw up in the nearest toilet. I haven't had a blood test since!'

For Jessie, then aged eleven, it was quite different: 'I was fascinated by mine. I watched the whole time as the thick, red liquid spilled into the glass vial.'

Typically, Jemma, then fourteen, took it all in her stride: 'I remember that each time we visited you there was always lots of laughter and smiles, it always felt positive. I can't remember ever feeling upset at seeing you in hospital.'

What Doc Oc and his team were looking for were similarities between certain sets of markers. Human leukocyte antigen (HLA) is a protein – aka a marker – found on most cells in your body. The best transplant outcomes are created when a patient's HLA and the donor's HLA closely match. Half of your HLA markers are inherited from your mother and half from your father. Each brother and sister has a 25%, or one in four, chance of matching if you have the same mother and father. It is highly unlikely that other family members will match with you. Under rare circumstances, family members other than siblings may be tested. About 70%, or seven out of ten, patients who need a transplant do not have a suitable donor in their family. In such cases, your transplant team will look for an unrelated donor. A search on The Bone Marrow Registry includes more than 22.5 million potential adult donors on lists collected from around the world. This sounds like a lot, but taking into account the criteria for a good match and the global population, the simple fact is: more donors are always needed.

There are many different HLA markers and each has a name. Doctors review at least eight HLA markers for these minimum requirements: two A markers, two B markers, two C markers, and two DRB1 markers. Some doctors look for an additional matching marker called DQ. An adult donor must match at least six of these eight HLA markers. Many transplant centres require at least seven out of eight matches before going ahead with the procedure.

Dr. Prem Mahendra is a Consultant Haemato-Oncologist at the Queen Elizabeth Hospital, Birmingham – henceforth referred to as the QE. She specialises in leukaemia, myeloma, and lymphoma. Prem had only been in her role for a couple of years when I became her patient, but in that short time had already set up a dedicated transplant unit that has since gone on to become one of the largest in the UK, with over 220 procedures performed each year. She is an indomitable force for good.

Completely rebuilt in 2006, the QE is now amongst the busiest single-site NHS hospitals in the UK, with over a thousand beds. During my stay in 2000, they were still coping with a charming mix of the very old and the very new. Original 18th century buildings stood beside curved modern towers and portacabins. A multi-floored maze of different departments and corridors lay inside.

We first met with Dr. Mahendra in late January at her day clinic, tucked away in the bowels of the sprawling complex. After a clinic nurse had taken my bloods, Mum, Dad, and I were shown into her makeshift office. The walls were painted a lurid blue.

Coming face-to-face with her brown, twinkling eyes and warm smile, I immediately felt in good hands. The fact she could switch from belly laughter to life-or-death seriousness in mere seconds endeared her to me, just as it had with Dr. O'Connor. Two dedicated and intelligent scientists who understood the importance of a healthy sense of humour. Prem wasted no time in getting to the heart of the matter:

'Jody, a bone marrow transplant is your best chance at a cure, but it is not without risk, you know. There is a 20% chance it won't be successful. I'm telling you this because you have to be prepared for that possibility. It depends very much on the match we get with your brother and sisters, who I believe are currently being tested,' she looked at Dad for confirmation.

'That's right,' he said.

'If we don't get a strong match with them we have to open it up to the public registers, and aside from being more unpredictable, that can take up valuable time.'

Despite Doc Oc's declaration that my cancer was in remission, and despite fighting off pneumonia and MRSA, I was once again reminded that death leered over my shoulder. Nothing was certain. Memories flashed up in my mind's eye: sobbing into Mum's jacket at Bridgnorth Surgery, the sensation of air being forced into my lungs as the rubber straps of the CPAP mask dug deep into my skin, the emotion on Tasha's face when she first saw me in the ICU.

I decided to place all my energy into that 80% chance. Those were still fucking good odds for anyone in my position. Of course I was onboard.

'So what happens next?' I said.

'As soon as we get the results back from your siblings' tests we'll bring you into the haematology ward. My secretary, Angela, will phone you within the next week and then we'll start preparing for treatment.'

That concluded our first meeting. I left feeling hopeful but scared shitless. This was make or break. Even though I'd made it through three months of hellish struggle into remission, I knew that the transplant had to be carried out. If I'd chosen to gamble by finishing my treatment early, the constant underlying worry about the leukaemia returning would likely have destroyed me.

Jessie and I have always been close, ever since she was small. As my littlest sister, I found her goofyness adorable. Her surreal sense of humour appealed to my own love of wordplay and the absurd. We are similar in many ways, although her diva-like tantrums made her the butt of a good few family in-jokes.

Amongst the four of us, bonds between two pairs naturally

formed. Jemma and Josh developed a strong bond, while Jessie and I did the same. It wasn't that I didn't feel deeply connected with my other siblings, far from it. Each connection brought different blessings and I valued them all individually. It was more that there was an ease to the communication between Jess and I which meant we just enjoyed hanging out and doing similar things.

After a tense period of wondering what the hell I would do if none of them were a match, the results finally came back. The plan was for me to stay at home for several weeks to rest and build strength whilst the donor situation was resolved. There had to be a match in place before I could be booked into the QE for my transplant. One afternoon Doc Oc called the house and asked for me, we chatted briefly and I hung up. Walking back into the lounge, Jessie was curled up on the sofa, her hand resting on the remote.

'So, Doc Oc says I've got to be very nice to you from now on...' I said casually from the doorway.

She glanced up from her TV show. 'Oh yeah, why's that then?'

'Be-cause... you're my match!'

Her face lit up and she dropped the remote. Leaping across the room she dived in to hug me, breaking out in a grin as the relief overflowed.

'And... it's not just that we match, he says you're a *perfect match* – isn't that incredible?'

'Oh Jode, that's amazing!' She started to cry. As we clasped each other tightly, I began to take in this new understanding that she could literally save me, that within my sister's bones may well be a lifeline.

'I knew it. I knew you'd be a match, Jess. Didn't we say just last week, if it was going to be anyone it was going to be you,' I was supercharged, glowing.

'I know!' she said, 'I felt like it was going to be me too, I can't explain it, I just knew,' her voice squeaked with excitement. 'You're going owe me,' she joked, prodding my chest.

'Ok, umm, how about a McDonald's when this is all over? My treat.'

She laughed at the deliberate inadequacy of the offer, fixed me with a practiced look of faux-seriousness. 'Sure, you're on.'

We embraced again. I knew it wasn't a surefire thing, that there was still a slight chance that the whole procedure could fail. But I didn't give that thought any power. I knew in my heart this was the miracle I needed. From that moment on, part of me knew I would survive. On that day of true hope, my smile shone out like a beacon high on a mountain top, visible far across the land. The rest of the family gathered around us to share the amazing news. There were hugs, tears and smiles. You could track the colour flowing back into my parents' faces. For the first time since my diagnosis, I could almost permit myself to relax, even if just for a couple of minutes. I hurried upstairs to my room to call Tash and share the good news.

Later, when the elation had died down, our parents explained to Jess that there was still a chance the transplant might not work, even with the strength of our match. 'If it doesn't work, you mustn't blame yourself,' Mum said.

Jessie recalls: 'I loved her for being that thoughtful, to try and prepare me beforehand, to see that I would have blamed myself. But to me, it didn't matter what she said. I was your only chance, and I was not going to let you down. If I had, I would have never forgiven myself or God. I started eating healthily. A wild friend offered me a cigarette which I turned down, telling her with grave solemnity, "I need to keep my blood healthy for Jody." And I've never told you this but for years after, and even now sometimes, I felt guilty when I ate something shit, or smoked, or drank too much. Not because I was worried for my own health, but because I knew that there might be a day when you'd need me again, and I didn't want to hurt your chances of recovery in the event of a relapse.'

Jemma remembers her own, very different reaction: 'I was actually really upset I wasn't a match. I'd thought it would be me, being the oldest sibling. Jess and I were going to do an assembly about the transplant, but she was unwell, so I took a photo of her and did the assembly on my own. My friends came over to listen and support me. We did some fundraising asking kids to put any spare change from lunch into a pot and we donated it to charity.'

Back at the hospital, these events had set everything in motion. Dr. Mahendra was delighted, her booming 'Haugh Haugh Haugh!' laughter filled the room on our next visit. For the doctors, this was the best possible outcome; such a match was very rare. It could only have been better if we were identical twins. That continues to astound me. It was, and still is, an emotionally-charged concept. It's high drama – the distilled essence of what it means to be part of a family – and a very beautiful thing. What were the chances that she would be born with exactly the right combination of cellular markers inside her bones? A combination that could save my life.

The transition from Shrewsbury over to the specialist unit at Birmingham was underway. After a series of visits to the outpatients department for preliminary checks, my admittance was scheduled for mid-February. On one of these reconnaissance trips, Prem asked to speak with Dad in private.

I wandered down to the lounge, a cosy space at the end of the corridor with large windows on three sides, providing a birds-eye view over the hospital roofs and grey Edgbaston streets to the city centre high-rises on the horizon. It was furnished with a couple of battered easy chairs, a brown laminated coffee table littered with old copies of magazines, and a full water cooler. I stood leaning my hands on the window ledge. The sun managed a pale winter sparkle. There is something magical in seeing things from a greater perspective than the everyday. It stirs my soul. I find a great sense of peace in quietly taking in all the details. I remained in silence for several minutes before the door opened and a middle-aged man stumbled in. He looked drunk. I was bemused. We stood side by side, staring out at sprawling, industrial Birmingham.

'Not bad eh? What you in for?' he said.

'I've got leukaemia,' I said. 'I'm here to arrange my transplant.'

'Oh right,' he said, looking me up and down. 'You know what's good for you then? Guinness. You need the iron man, I'm telling you. A few cans every day, it'll fix you right up. Full of iron. It's medicine, man.'

I laughed nervously.

'You think I'm joking? I'm not joking,' he said, his voice rising.

'Maybe I'll give that a go,' I said, lying politely.

'Yeah you should, good luck to you mate, alright, cool, look after yourself, see you around,' he replied hazily, wandering off to find a trashy magazine. He slumped himself in one of the easy chairs with his feet up on the coffee table.

Amongst the vast glossary of complex medical terminology I'd heard throughout my treatment, there was always something very distinctive about the word 'transplant'. It carries a range of strongly defined emotions and opinions. It describes the addition of something external into one's own body. An upgrade. A futuristic and mysterious operation, it conjures images of nanotechnology and biomechanical engineering, dead people's kidneys, lungs, and even pig's hearts saving lives. It's a scary but unmistakably exciting procedure, another chance at life when a vital part of you is malfunctioning or shutting down. We can already see the near-future of lab-grown organs, developed from our own stem cells to ensure bodily rejections are kept to an absolute minimum.

Most people don't fully understand what a bone marrow transplant actually is. I sure didn't, and I probably still don't. I'd seen the animal bones happily gnawed upon for hours in the back garden by Mac, our family's Golden Retriever, and I had a vague awareness that the gloopy, pinky-red stuff inside them was marrow. With my newfound haematology knowledge, I understood that the bone marrow was where the immature cells, known to us as stem cells, are produced. In fact, most blood cells in the body develop in the bone marrow, producing more than 200 billion new ones every single day. Mightily impressive.

So what actually happens? The first stage is to prepare the patient's body for the transplant with a strong dose of chemotherapy. This is called *conditioning* and is done to kill any remaining cancer cells that might be hiding in the body, even if the cancer has been declared 'in remission', as mine had. It also resets the patient's immune system to a level where the body is not as able to fight the foreign cells. The possibility of rejection is the main concern with many kinds of transplants and is usually managed with specialised drugs. With bone marrow transplants especially, lowering immunity is essential as the process involves sowing the seeds for a brand new immune system to grow. It also clears out any old stem cells in the marrow to make way for the donated ones.

For the donor, the main event is the extraction of the bone marrow itself and is usually completed over the course of a single day. After being admitted to hospital, they be will taken to theatre and given anaesthetic. The surgeon uses a special hollow needle to withdraw marrow from the back of the pelvis. As they recover, it's common for the donor to receive a blood transfusion of their own previously collected blood. The donor may feel stiff and sore around the area for up to a week afterwards. If the extraction is not delivered on the same day, the marrow must be frozen along with a preservative, which can sometimes cause additional side-effects for the recipient.

Once the transplant patient has completed the conditioning process and their neutrophils are low enough, the second stage of the transplant can take place, where the donor's fresh bone marrow is delivered intravenously through the Hickman line. At this point the patient is extremely vulnerable, having no immune system. For both the conditioning and the transplant itself, the patient must be isolated in a sealed room that cannot be entered from outside without passing through an 'air lock' system. Everyone must follow a strict protocol of cleansing their hands and donning aprons, gloves, and face masks. This all felt pretty severe pre-Covid. As with my previous rounds of chemo, visitors or staff with any hint of a cough, cold, or skin condition were not allowed in. The risks are too great – the slightest infection could be fatal.

Then finally, all that's left to do is wait as the donated stem cells do their job, endure the chemo side-effects, and hope that the body does not reject the foreign cells.

Part Three

SOLVE ET COAGULA

Pain is a holy angel which has brought humans more gnosis than joy ever could.

Adalbert Stifter,
Austrian theologist

Ω

The Bone Collector

The old woman reached for her battered sheepskin jacket and slipped it on. This one dropped past her knees and once buttoned-up, swaddled her completely. Stitched onto the front and sides were woven pockets of varying sizes. Crumbs of wood and loam in one, sandy grit in another. In the breast pocket, a scrap of dried meat sat twisted and half-chewed. Patting herself down she retrieved the morsel, sniffed it with three short huffs. Having decided it was edible, she gnawed at her stashed treat, perching on a stool to pull on her boots.

As the sun kissed the horizon, granting dusk a stage, she took her leather satchel and a walking stick, left the cabin, and trudged off in a north-westerly direction. To the untrained eye the landscape was amorphous, no tree different from the next. But this wise one held the landscape within her, mapped out on the scrolls of her

ancient mind. She knew the invisible pathways that ran across the
scrub and could follow the tracks of deer, rat, and wolf. She joined
the arroyo that snaked off westwards as she had done a thousand
times before.

Following the twists and turns of this sleeping waterway, the
old crone made her way deep into the heart of the desert until the
riverbed came to an end at the foot of a slope. As she walked, she
hummed a timeless, looping melody. The distant mountains drifted
slowly out of focus as daylight began to fade.

There was a reason for being out here on this walkabout. Her
intent was to search for bones. Not just any bones. The bones of
a wolf. She paused to rest and listen. To truly listen. The howling
echoes called to her. From her handcrafted satchel, she pulled out
a heavy torch with a handle on its topside, scanning the ground as
she walked.

Engaging all her senses, *La Trapera*, the gatherer, started to hunt
for wolf bones. The pack lived in and around these foothills and
she knew the places where they went to die. Her melody shifted,
changed, and then stopped. Wandering on in silence, broad beams of
light washed across the terrain, seeking the glimmer of a fragment.
The moon was not yet new. It hung secretly in the sky, waiting for
its moment to shine.

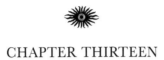

CHAPTER THIRTEEN

Shifting Seasons

February was fading fast and the light of March was just starting to show. I could almost feel the first warm breezes blowing fresh spring air. It had been a long hard winter, the hardest and longest of my life. I'd made it back from the brink of death's wide-open door in intensive care, thanks in part to my murderous dream hit-squad. I fought with all I had, managing to stay mindfully engaged. I trusted the process, accepting the destructive chemicals, the radiation and the injections, allowing it all in.

What mattered now was that my cancer was in remission. The cancer cells were undetectable in my blood, but crucially this did not mean they'd all been cleared. Some could be hiding within my organs or tucked away inside my bones. Tricksters, waiting in the shadows until it all went quiet, until no-one would suspect a thing, only to leap out and restart their destructive campaign of rapid division once more.

The bone marrow transplant was on. A magnificent gift from my bloodline, Jessie's body held exactly what mine needed. Back at the family home in Bridgnorth, she was preparing for her own journey of donation. In a couple of weeks, when Prem decided the time was right, Jessie would be whisked off to Birmingham Children's Hospital to have a small amount of bone marrow removed from her pelvis.

I was to spend my first couple of days at the QE on the haematology ward, receiving the regulatory bags of blood, platelets, saline, and of course, a cocktail of different drugs. Once my isolation room was ready, I'd be moved in and the high-dose conditioning chemo would commence. After a period of rest, allowing my body to detox the drugs, Jessie's fresh bone marrow cells would be delivered into my bloodstream. And after that? Weeks of waiting.

On the day I arrived on the ward, a young South Asian lad lay on the next bed. His skin had turned a striking shade of yellow. A custardy shade of yellow coloured his face, spreading out across the rest of his body. I'd never seen anything like it. Apparently, his liver had been greatly affected by his condition and he was struggling. Our eyes met in silent recognition. He looked at me like a crab peering out from beneath its shell. I lay down on the bed and Mum busied herself, setting up my bedside table with everything I'd need. After a while, several members of his family arrived, four or

five people, and they began to share a feast of Indian food. Dishes
kept appearing from various bags and they all sat around and ate
together, although the lad barely touched anything his Dad fed him.
The pungent aroma was quite overwhelming for me as my sense of
smell was a little out of kilter and the fumes wafting from the next
bed quickly made me feel nauseous. Mum was about to get up and
have a quiet word but one of the nurses clocked me struggling and
the feast was grumpily packed away to be resumed in the privacy
of the day lounge down the hall.

The ward was fairly small, with only eight beds. It had a couple
of private rooms too, but the large isolation room where I'd be
heading was further up the corridor, near the main nurse's office.
These were specifically built for patients undergoing a bone marrow
transplant.

After a couple of days, Kate, the BMT nurse, came to let me
know that I could move in to my new room later that afternoon.
They were just finishing off the deep clean. As I approached the
door my body tingled. I was stepping into this place for a period of
several weeks and would not be allowed out. Very few people would
be allowed in. This was it. Showtime. With all the anticipation, I
could have been walking out to the ring at Madison Square Garden,
or heading through the backstage tunnels towards the main stage
at Wembley Arena. It was quite the rush. A couple of breaths and
an internal pep-talk outside the doors and in we went.

The room was a good size with a cosy living space set up beyond
the sleeping area. There was a chest of drawers for my things, a
small sofa and a couple of easy chairs. A TV with VHS player, a CD
player, a kettle, and a fridge. Up on the back wall was a window. It

was too high for me to look out of but allowed in a good amount of natural light. The bathroom was a kind of ensuite; a small plastic-coated pod built into a hole in the wall. You just opened a door and stepped right in. My room was certainly comfortable and I felt happy to see out the procedure there. The other isolation room next door became home to the Indian boy who I'd seen on my first day. Every now and then I noticed a member of his family coming and going through his air lock doors.

> **From:** Tash
> **Sent:** 07:33 am
> Hope you're settling in ok gorgeous,
> I'll come over as soon as I can. Love T xxx

Though I was now a couple of hours drive away from Bridgnorth, Tasha still came to visit and we'd chat on the phone every few days. She was focusing on her A-levels, preparing for the upcoming exams, as well as part-time waitressing at a pub in the town. Tash looked tired. The poor girl had been on quite a journey with me over the past three months.

Quite coincidentally, her Dad's business, a prestige gunmaking firm, lay within walking distance of the hospital grounds. When she could, she'd hop a lift into Birmingham with him and head over to see me. Beneath her usual confidence, I could tell she was nervous about the procedure I was about to go through. She would never have said it to my face, but the look in her eyes spoke loud and clear.

'Almost there, Jode, I know you can do it.' She took my hand and squeezed it.

The proclamation that my leukaemia was in remission had created a kind of false finale; yes you're better, but… In a case like mine, reaching remission didn't really carry the same sense of celebration that it would for other kinds of cancer. The doctors and I were aiming for a cure, nothing less. By now I was now well aware of the 20% failure rate, and all the risks and complications surrounding a bone marrow transplant. If for any reason my body rejected Jessie's stem cells I could die. That was certainly a potential outcome, and while it did scare me to a degree, I was bubbling with a kind of nervous excitement for the first time in months.

I had the sense I'd already come as close to death as I was going to get. Drifting between states of consciousness – especially during the monumental events of my morphine dreams – had changed me. Emboldened, I believed I had survived for a reason. I didn't yet comprehend the gifts afforded me during that time and was still coming to terms with the sheer magic of it all. In my mind, I was walking the winding road back home, despite understanding the possibility that further risks lay ahead.

Jessie being my match was a miracle that I trusted. The risk of failure didn't worry me as much as it might have if I'd had a non-family donor, or if the match hadn't been quite as perfect. I made a promise to myself: if I got through this final trial, I'd be forever grateful, never taking for granted what a precious gift it is to simply be alive.

I lay in my spotless isolation room contemplating all the unbelievable trials I'd been put through to get to this point. Gradually, my awareness settled on a tiny golden seed somewhere inside me.

It spoke of hope and an unfailing belief in my body's survival. At the core of this seed lay a potent energy I can only describe as pure life force. If I was still and quiet, I could just about feel it radiating throughout my body. It called to me, asking me to listen.

The conditioning chemo had begun and I could feel what little reserves of strength I'd stockpiled during January swiftly melt away. One morning after breakfast, I stood underneath the scalding water and looked up. There, above my head, was a small light. For some reason it caught my eye, and I decided to try a spontaneous experiment. Closing my eyes, I visualised a pure ray of light flowing down from miles above me, pouring into and around my body. In my mind's eye, I pictured the source as a vast white lake. A stream of this liquid light flowed into the showerhead, infusing every droplet. The charged water soaked my skin, moving through my body from my crown all the way down to my feet, as I gave the practice all the concentration I could muster.

After some time had passed, I stopped the shower. My body was calm, my muscles relaxed, I was a little lightheaded perhaps, but my mind was clear. 'What the hell was that?' I mumbled to myself with a half-smile. I wasn't quite sure where it had come from or how it worked but that didn't worry me. Whatever I'd just done had made a dramatic difference. I felt so grounded and at ease I actually laughed out loud with joy. Who knew what effect it might have had on my physical body?

I decided to repeat the method every morning for as long as I could. It gave me a strength I could draw on without depleting myself. Very much the opposite in fact – it felt nourishing. I hadn't done anything like this before, or ever read about such a technique, and yet my experience said: this works. That is a rule I have tried to live by ever since; if it works for you then it works, and don't let anyone tell you otherwise.

Thanks to the pioneering work of Dr. Candace Pert – who you may remember from Chapter Seven – we know that our feelings and emotions directly effect our cells at the molecular level, and can consequently impact disease outcomes. *Scientific American* reports that the reward circuit which I unknowingly triggered with my shower meditation has been shown to reach the immune system and empower a subset of bone marrow cells, even slowing the growth of tumours. Although this study was conducted on mice rather than humans, it promises to provide validating evidence of the mind's ability to affect the physical health of the body.

Given that the reward system is linked with positive emotions, this research offers a physiological mechanism for how a person's mental state could help stall the progression of cancer. This is so fucking exciting I feel the need to swear. This is endo-immuno-therapy – a self-generated immune response to fight off disease.

As you might expect, the mice researchers found that chronic emotional stress also targets the same cells. Deeply negative feelings can have a negative impact on the immune system and actually reduce its effectiveness against diseases like cancer. The importance of addressing the stress which pervades our modern lives can therefore not be overstated. There is a hell of a lot we can do preventatively if only we can take a step back from the daily grind and prioritise our mental, physical, and spiritual health.

In his landmark book *The Brain That Changes Itself*, Norman Doidge describes how via the science of neuroplasticity it is possible for our thoughts to actually change the structure and function of our brains. The brain is not a static system, but rather something that has the potential to re-organise itself. This is a radical understanding. In the book, Doidge cites miraculous patient recovery stories, such as a stroke patient who learns to speak again and a woman born with half a brain that rewires itself to function as a whole.

Neuroplasticity provides evidence that the brain has a capacity for healing and adaptation that is beyond all previous conceptions. Imagine then, what may be possible for those who apply this dormant power to the rest of the body.

After a couple of days, I once again felt battered by the chemo. They'd given me several bags and the now-familiar effects began in earnest; I was shitting water every thirty minutes, often throwing up during the same trip to the toilet. The colour had drained from my face and I was losing the energy to even get out of bed. It took a heroic effort to even roll over during the night.

I was quite lucky with sleep, managing without too much disturbance other than the odd 3 am toilet mission. The extra drugs I was on to control the side-effects were working, meaning that while I did suffer, it could have been so much worse. I still had no hair on my entire body. As a skinny bald boy, I now resembled my teenage hero, Smashing Pumpkins frontman Billy Corgan, a resemblance not lost to my friend, Rob, when out for a drink to celebrate my remission a few weeks prior. Gentle ribbing is healthy, a bit of banter between friends was something I'd missed a great deal. A little taste of everyday life, back in the world I felt a million miles removed from.

As my body slowed down and the impact of the chemo grew stronger, I struggled to keep on top of it. I slept a lot. When I was awake I was increasingly bored, losing interest in listening to music and reading. The TV was on for background noise most of the time. Mum and Dad alternated their visits, occasionally bringing my siblings along. The image of them dutifully putting on their plastic aprons and gloves stuck with me; they looked like a little team of child cleaners on their first day at work.

The nurses took a stool sample from me every day. By that I mean I defecated in a small kidney-shaped cardboard box and handed it over. Underneath the main window was a cupboard with sliding doors on both sides – a hatch to place my shit receptacle for the nurses to retrieve in their own time and without having to enter the room.

My BMT nurse was a twinkly-eyed lady named Kate. As far as I could tell, the others were agency staff who worked to a rota I could never quite figure out. Due to lack of contact I didn't get to know any of them to the same degree as Luanne, Emma, and Mary. Nevertheless, I found them to be devoted and patient human beings. They'd joke and smile with me, and bring fresh jugs of iced water. The team were much busier than in Shrewsbury, with more patients to attend to and more comings and goings; there wasn't much time for the sort of one-to-ones I'd been lucky to have before. The atmosphere on the ward felt brusker too, more serious. Everyone seemed to have somewhere to be. For the most part, I didn't mind, it focused me on the task at hand. They had a job to do and so did I.

At Shrewsbury, by the time they brought the food trolley round it was generally lukewarm and unsurprisingly average – overcooked and under-seasoned. The QE, despite being a much larger hospital with hundreds of mouths to feed, faired better in this department. With so many South Asian patients there were plenty of fragrant curries, but everything just tasted bland. The chemo had nuked my appetite again too. I sometimes snacked on a few handfuls of crisps and fruit when I felt able. Mum would bring me Fox's Glacier mints to take the edge off my horrendously sore dry-mouth, which at times felt like it was lined with sawdust.

I had asked for a Nintendo Gameboy that Christmas. These days they have been resigned to the archives of video gaming history, but around the turn of the century they were all the rage. It was all I wanted. I needed a way to keep my brain engaged and my mind distracted, and I had the feeling that a game like *Tetris* would do the trick.

Throughout my teens, my parents had steadfastly rejected games consoles, much to my continued annoyance. When the Sega Megadrive and the Super Nintendo came blasting onto the scene, Sonic the Hedgehog spinning his spiky blue mane across magazines and TV adverts, every kid wanted in. The latest games and highest scores were popular topics of conversation on the playground. Yet however much I moaned and groaned, Mum and Dad stood firm. I guess they didn't want me sat in front of the TV every night, glued to *Super Mario Brothers*, and I can understand that. Instead, I poured all my spare time into practising drums until we finally got a family PC and I discovered the zombie-blasting delights of *Doom*.

Now I had a Gameboy. It wasn't quite the eye-popping 16-bit psychedelia of the big consoles, but at least I could call myself a gamer, earning me some street-cred back at school. The yellow handheld console came with a couple of games: *The Legend of Zelda* and *Tetris*. Sat up in bed or on the easy chairs when I was able, I'd zone out in 3D block land. Mum sat opposite, reading her book or listening to the radio, pausing occasionally to ask me to turn the volume down as that famously hummable soundtrack pumped from its tiny speaker.

After a week of intravenous chemotherapy, I was totally wiped out. It was a Friday and I was given several days off just to rest. The bone marrow transplant had been arranged for the following Monday. Jessie was booked into Birmingham Children's Hospital and the stage was set. The mythology of the story we were living hung suspended in the air. Prem had been round to tell us she was happy to initiate the process, providing my blood results were satisfactory. Shivers washed through me as nervous excitement swirled. *This is really happening. Happening to me.* The isolation room could have drawn my story to an end, becoming my final resting place. Instead, it shaped my salvation.

A key ingredient of any positive mindset is the ability to separate any expectation of the eventual outcome from the fierce determination it takes to push towards what you want. It sounds paradoxical, but it's vital to accept all potential outcomes without drowning in fear or floating off on a cloud of pure hope. In Buddhism, this is known as non-attachment, which is often our greatest challenge, especially when facing events that terrify us. I find this fascinating, particularly the concepts surrounding fear. American mythologist Michael Meade ventures deep into this topic on his consistently excellent *Living Myth* podcast, as well as in his essays and articles. Meade writes:

> *'Fears arise wherever people face the unknown, whenever they feel unprotected and experience a serious loss of control in their lives. An old proverb warns that, "Those who live in fear can only live a half-life." Fear itself is a natural emotion, an inner stirring of instincts and intuitions that can include our deepest survival resources. Healthy fear involves a sudden increase of awareness that can be life-protective and even life-saving.'*

From my understanding, fear is neither good nor bad, healthy nor unhealthy, it is simply a physiological response. Feeling fear is not a choice. However, our reaction to fear can be, depending upon our resources – experiences lived, witnessed, or heard; support, physiology, and health – and our ability to access them.

It's a complex subject, one that is often over-rationalised and misconstrued. *Feel the fear and do it anyway* – wildly empowering for some yet dangerously coercive for others. Impending fear may have greater negative impact than the fearful event itself, as you are constantly needing to overcome it until it actually happens, hence why many struggle with anxiety. I can only speak of my own experiences and what works for me, exploring such concepts from where I am today, but by approaching fear from the angle of curiosity over despair I have discovered strategies which positively impact my life.

When overcome by fear, our self-belief is suppressed. This feeling of powerlessness is extremely debilitating. A lack of personal power means we are unable to stand up for ourselves and take ownership of a situation. Fear creates a prison in the mind.

Interestingly, the etymology of the word fear can be traced back to the word *fare*, meaning thoroughfare: a journey, passage, or pathway. Meade surmises that fear, therefore, indicates what we must undergo, what must be faced, entered, and followed all the way through. In his words: *our greatest fears mark the thoroughfares where our souls would have us go*. Facing our fears is perhaps one of our greatest challenges as a species. Finding the path, the thoroughfare, between the extremes of being immobilised by fear and the denial of its existence is a balancing act. Both places deplete happiness. Once we have a handle on the 'healthy' aspects of our fear, we find we have a greater choice.

In the depths of fear, hope shines a light. Hope is a leap into the unknown, a step taken with trust. As Nelson Mandela said, '*hope is a powerful weapon, even when all else is lost.*' It is a letting go of what we are resisting, remaining open to the nowness of our experience – that place of infinite potential where anything can happen. Letting go, for me, meant an unconscious attempt to move beyond the dualism of whether I lived or died. For my own happiness, I could not risk being so attached. Accepting all aspects of my situation gave me the power to choose how I lived in each moment.

This is the same state that Tibetan Buddhist writer and teacher Chögyam Trungpa introduced in *Shambhala: The Sacred Path of the*

Warrior, a book published two years after my birth in 1984. By following the discipline of warriorship, and in particular the skill of
letting go, one can discover a bank of self-existing energy that is
always available, beyond any circumstance. The Tibetans call this
energy *lungta*, or windhorse. *Lung* meaning wind and *ta* meaning horse.

Trungpa taught that the cultivation of a warrior mindset incor-
porates skills such as the synchronisation of mind and body, as
well as the ability to relax within discipline. Facing the world with
openness and fearlessness. It is here we can discover the sacred in
amongst the noise of everyday life.

When I read this book years after my experience, I lit up. Here
was a spiritual teacher describing the kind of warrior I felt I had
to become while living through leukaemia. There were immediate
and obvious parallels with the way I'd intuitively approached my
acute dilemma. Without knowing what I was doing, I recognised
that I was, at times, able to touch the state of being that Trungpa
calls *unconditional confidence*. Not having confidence in something,
but settling into the feeling of confidence; an unwavering state of
mind that needs no reference point.

Trungpa described the kind of person I really wanted to be and
it created an ideal to aspire to. He outlined the qualities I wished to
emulate. The central concept is that once the warrior has discovered
the essence of sacredness within each moment, the beauty beneath
all life, they can radiate it out into the world for the good of all; a
kind of service that requires a little effort, yet ultimately bestows
great rewards.

Ω

The Hunt

On her altar in the cabin, she already had a wolf skull complete with a jaw, a tail, and many ribs. She had toe digits, a humerus, and pieces of backbone, but she didn't yet have everything. For the ceremony, she needed a complete skeleton. Before the work could begin she had to continue the hunt. Duty compelled her but she never once complained. She understood the work and went about it with a softness of heart and a complete dedication to her craft.

Her mind was still, the distractions of petty thoughts happily absent. From the moment she left the cabin she had entered a state that some call the warrior-mind; a ceremonial synchronisation of mind and body. Clarity of intent guided her walking feet as her open heart received and responded to new slivers of information.

Flitting her torch beam amongst some rocks, the light presented a glinting clue. She wandered over and knelt down in the dirt, dug a little. It was a pelvis. She placed it into her bag. More bones would surely be close by. A short distance away she found a patella with the femur still partly attached. Each time she discovered a fragment of the skeleton, be it a rib, a fibula, or a section of vertebrae, she muttered a short prayer and placed it into her satchel. After some time she had almost everything she needed.

Night had fallen. Clouds obscured the stars. She could smell the animals that thrived best after dark, they too were out to hunt and forage, making their way in the world. The last bones to be found were a pair of large shins, the tibia. One had splintered and the drying marrow was visible. No doubt that those dark red cells once lived inside a deer or a coyote. Life eats life and the wolf was no different.

The collection had been made, the bones were ready. Her satchel bulged with its weighty cargo. The chirruping song of a Chuck-will's-widow split the silence. She took it as a sign to return to the cabin, back to the warmth of the fire. At the trunk of a nearby tree, she placed an offering, a bundle of various herbs, semi-precious stones, and foods that she had picked out and wrapped before leaving. Together they represented her gratitude. It was her way of giving thanks for what she had found, a mark of respect to the spirits of the wolf, and the desert. Reciprocation is the proper way of things.

Satisfied, she began the walk home, re-tracing her steps down the gritty slopes and along the wandering arroyo, using her stick for balance. There was magic in the night air, each moment pregnant with opportunity. She revelled in this feeling as she walked and wondered if she would ever tire of it.

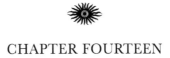

CHAPTER FOURTEEN

My Sister's Bones

With her best shoes on, a cute little dress and a shiny clutch bag, Jessie strutted proudly into Birmingham Children's Hospital, ready to donate in style. Determined to give of herself to help her big brother. All the nurses thought it was impossibly sweet.

The transplant procedure was set for the following day. They'd asked her to fast for twelve hours so she spent the evening on her bed chatting to Dad and reading. Some of the kids on the ward were in heartbreaking states and cries could be heard throughout the night. The next morning, after a few more hours of waiting around, the anaesthetist finally called her in.

Dad held her hand as they wheeled her down to the operating room.

'Sweet dreams, darling,' he whispered, as the injection flooded her body with temporary unconsciousness, the world fading to black in front of her eyes.

In the midst of the procedure, whilst floating through silver clouds, she awoke.

'Jessie, stop moving,' a voice said firmly.

It took her a few moments to realise her body was shaking uncontrollably. In an instant the anaesthetic-induced shivering stopped as everything went dark once more. Four hours later, she woke to the sight of Dad's worried face. She felt sick and dizzy.

'Did it go ok?' she asked.

'It went perfectly, Jess,' he assured.

I was in the shower when Mum arrived. Nervously, I dried off. While I was getting dressed, Mum updated me on Jessie's experience. In that very moment we sat there talking, my little sister was lying prone in an operating theatre on the other side of the city. We marvelled over her. My heart surged with love. It must have taken real courage to step up to something like this. She was a strong kid and my hope was that this experience would make her stronger still.

After a couple of long and anxious hours, there was a sudden flurry of activity. Two porters arrived and parked a trolley outside my room. The nurses on duty were expecting them and sprang into action. Soon, Kate was hooking up my drip and flushing my line with saline. The porters wheeled in what I can only describe as a festival-sized coolbox.

'Well Jody, this is your sister's bone marrow!' Kate said.

She flipped open the cooler and fished out a transparent bag filled with thick, pinkish goo. Apart from the colour, it looked remarkably similar to the bags of other people's blood I'd received during the course of treatment. I almost felt a bit let down. Seriously… was that it? This tiny bag of jelly was the healing miracle that could save my life? Yet that was exactly what it was: a pinkish bag of miracles. The cure to my disease hung right there before us.

I began to process what was happening, shifting rapidly from an initial sense of nonchalance to the brink of overwhelm. What an utter privilege it was to be a recipient of Jessie's freshly harvested cells. Kate attached it to my IV stand and hooked it up. I watched in awe as it drip, drip, dripped down the translucent, snaking tube and entered my bloodstream. Knowing that this substance had been hidden away inside the very core of my sister's bones just a few hours before blew my mind. Tingles of emotion zipped through me.

Mum and I sat and took in its humble, gravity-powered journey, both moved by the spectacle, both hoping upon hope that my body would welcome the goo to its new home. I was to have two bags of these stem cells. Within an hour one was inside me. By lunchtime, it was all done. The first phase of my transplant was over.

'What happens now?' I asked, incredulous at the painless simplicity.

Kate turned to us, her face professionally neutral. 'Now we just have to wait.'

The internal process following a BMT is really quite magical, pleasingly mysterious. Even today, I don't fully understand how it all works. What is clear to me, however, is that it demonstrates the incredible efficiency and miraculous nature of the human organism.

We are astoundingly well made. When Jessie's cells flowed into my bloodstream, quite remarkably they knew where to go and what to do.

They make their way steadily into the hosts' bones, taking root in the remains of the previously obliterated marrow. Ideally, they settle down in their new home and start to produce fresh stem cells, which will subsequently develop into healthy red and white blood cells. These fresh blood cells spread around the body, populating every vein, vessel, and organ, literally replenishing and revitalising the entire system.

The initial risk in all this is that the host body could view them as a foreign substance and might attack. If the host does have trouble accepting the cells, a series of symptoms are produced, diagnosed as Graft-versus-host-disease – GVHD. This can happen with any kind of transplant in any body. For some, it can be fatal, as the body flat-out rejects the transplant matter in what is known as a graft failure. Those with the best type of match may avoid GVHD all together, but most people do experience a mild case, often characterised by rashes on the hands and feet and accompanied by nausea and diarrhoea. It's a fairly normal physiological response and can even be considered a good thing as the donor T-cells work to kill off any remaining cancer cells. In any case, doctors are prepared with doses of a powerful anti-rejection drug called cyclosporin, which is derived from fungus.

This next phase would be hyper-critical to my survival. With no immune system and barely any white cells, a tiny infection could finish me off in no time. This was perhaps the most dangerous part of the entire treatment and the reason why they kept me isolated.

I'd read the sheet with a list of the likely side-effects but hadn't given it too much attention. It talked of a wide range of sympto-matic responses: fever and flushing, sudden pains in the chest and the body, headaches, diarrhoea, nausea and vomiting, shortness of breath, hives, and a strange taste in the mouth. I'd experienced almost all of these already in response to the chemo and radiotherapy, so for the most part I knew how to navigate them.

The other major concern was the potential for complications. Internal bleeding, damage to the kidneys, liver, lungs, and heart, inflammation, and damage to the stomach and digestive system – the rather grim list went on and on. I decided to try and stay as present as I could with whatever was happening. Mouth sores? Ok, we'll deal with them. Aches and pains? Fine, take your painkillers and try to move around the room a little. Keeping myself strong with whatever courage I could muster in the face of the unknown was my only option.

I was monitored closely. It was knife-edge time. I was instructed to honestly and openly report how I was feeling several times a day. If anything caused me specific discomfort, I should alert the nurses. Through blood, urine, and stool analysis, there were mechanisms in place to reduce the likelihood and potential impact of any side effects.

After the first twenty-four hours, I began to feel distinctly odd. I had intense night sweats and pulsating muscle aches. Shimmering nerve pains would pop up in different parts of my body and then disappear as if they'd never been there at all. My mouth broke out in stinging sores so now my food was mostly in liquid form. I often had loose stools and bouts of dizziness. When I needed something, I'd press the little red buzzer next to the bed and tell the nurses, who'd quickly return with the appropriate pills.

My body was out of whack. I imagined the chaos – messages firing from all directions at once along the spaghetti junction of my body. I was well aware of the tightrope-walking this process entailed, but just to make sure I understood the fragile nature of my predicament, I was given a stark reminder.

A few days post-transplant there had been a steady rotation of visitors to the other isolation room. Occasionally when my curtains were open, I caught a glimpse of the comings and goings in the corridor outside. When I asked what was going on, Kate told me that the South Asian boy with the yellow skin that I'd seen on my first day on the ward was next door. He was sick and struggling. They told me not to worry. He had undergone the transplant procedure via a donation from a member of the public on the Bone Marrow Register a week or so before my own. Over the course of the day he had more visitors, who I took to be members of his extended family. They all left looking ashen-faced.

The following night I was woken by a commotion. The unmistakable sound of a woman wailing drifted through the walls in the dirty half-light. I could feel the pain in her cry. This outpouring of grief continued for the next few hours. Steadily, more people came by. I heard more crying and screaming, then what sounded like chanting. I felt terrible for the family and what they must have been going through.

When I was woken by the nurses for breakfast, they gently told me that the boy had died just before dawn. Many members of his family had stayed with the body for a while afterwards, singing, praying, shouting their grievances to their gods. An older woman, who I assumed to be his mother, was inconsolable as she eventually left the room, weeping and remonstrating all the way out and down the corridor, supported by a group of family members.

Mum was visiting that day. She had walked by his family on the way in to see me and immediately understood what had happened. It affected her deeply. With a slight twist of fate, it could just as easily have been her son's life. She came in with eyes wet and shining, trying to stay strong for me but struggling. We spoke about it for a couple of minutes before she swiftly changed the subject. I understood, I didn't want to dwell on my possible demise either. The doctors had warned us about graft failure, but only with the boy's death did the risks now feel real. We accepted that this could happen to me, but my situation was also quite different. I was in much better health when I came in, having been in remission and with a month of rest behind me. I had my sister's well-matched bone marrow, which was one hell of a weapon – I refused to lose faith just because the same procedure had failed for someone else.

Since starting treatment, I'd not really stopped to think about the act of receiving while it was happening. I was always grateful, but saw the infusions of blood and platelets as simply part of the protocol. I didn't stop to question the origins of those bags of burgundy. Inevitably, one detaches from reality somewhat. Individual survival comes sharply into focus while everything else blends into a silky and unimportant background blur.

Reflecting on it now, I feel a surge of overwhelming gratitude to those dear selfless folks who donated their blood when I needed it so urgently. I wonder about their faces. Who were they? To think these people are walking around each day and I will never know them, never be able to hug or shake hands with them, nor offer a pint and conversation. If you've ever donated blood, sincerely, thank you. It's such a vital gift you have given. If you want to give blood, please don't put it off. Go ahead and schedule it in. There will always be someone in need.

Undergoing any form of transplant strikes me as an extremely intimate experience. I'd even suggest it is one of the most intimate experiences a human being can have. In taking a substance from the core of my sister's bones directly into my main artery, I received the essence of her being, the essential building blocks of her entire system.

Having incorporated Jessie's bone marrow, her specific sequencing of DNA now runs alongside my own. Medically speaking, this means that I have two sets of DNA, the codes to create two individual organisms. My blood DNA is identical to Jessie's, yet the DNA profile of the rest of my cells is, or perhaps was, still resolutely my own. Isn't that incredible? How miraculous to think that her blood flows in my veins as I weave my way through life. This rare process has forever linked us at the biological level as well as, I feel, the energetic, or what science now refers to as the quantum: that which lays underneath daily reality like a kind of universal base layer.

Of course, she had not taken in any of my DNA, yet through this transplant, through this entire experience, our sibling connection grew undeniably stronger in weird and wonderful ways. I see the transplant procedure as nothing less than an initiation ceremony for both of us, and to an extent, for our family and those around us. For a young girl on the brink of puberty, courageously allowing the extraction of her bone marrow must be a peak life experience. The nature of life and the inevitability of death are heavy topics for any eleven-year-old to get to grips with. The weight of giving your sibling another chance at life is immense, yet Jessie strode on in there and did what she had to do without complaining, without so much as a second thought. Jess tells me that the experience imprinted her with deep and lasting emotions that she'll carry throughout the rest of her days.

In classical Greek mythology there exists a creature composed of different kinds of DNA. Portrayed as a terrifying monster, the Chimera is a female amalgamation of a fire-breathing lion, a milk-laden goat, and a vicious serpent. The legend is thought to have originated as a deification of the volcano at Mount Chimera in modern-day Turkey, and the visual form influenced by lioness hybrids of earlier civilisations, such as the Egyptian diety Sekhmet, and the neo-Hittite Chimera of Carchemish. Along with other powerful female 'monsters' in the Greek pantheon such as Medusa, Scylla and Charybdis, the Chimera was likely created out of male fears around the power of females.

In *Women and Other Monsters: Building a New Mythology*, writer Jess Zimmerman points out that 'Women have been monsters, and monsters have been women, in centuries' worth of stories, because stories are a way to encode these expectations and pass them on.' Female monsters represent 'the bedtime stories patriarchy tells itself', reinforcing expectations about women's bodies and behaviour.

I remember the Chimera from a treasured book of myths and legends that I read as a child but it held no major significance. Only in recent years when learning that the word chimera also refers to a 'mixing of different forms' did I make the connection.

Sharing DNA with another human is highly unusual and I'd never considered what that entailed. It was only after a series of failed genome analysis tests with two of the most well-known companies that I began to question. AncestryDNA was able to shed some light on my failed reading:

> *'If you have received a bone marrow (or a stem cell transplant for that matter, too), your AncestryDNA test may provide unexpected results because your saliva may contain cells with your DNA as well as cells with your donor's DNA. DNA for the test is extracted from the cells, and the combination of DNA sources can result in a failed test or a test that provides results based on your donor's DNA. Therefore, we recommend that those who have received bone marrow do not take the test.'*

They seemed to be saying that mine and Jessie's DNA have combined into a form that is unreadable as a single DNA chain by their technology.

I am a chimera – the modern medical term given to a genetic hybrid with more than one set of DNA, in my case human male and human female. How this rare condition affects people like me has, to my knowledge, never been studied, but I think about it often. Have I taken on aspects of my sister? If so, what parts of her unique being did I somehow assimilate? Are the feminine aspects of my personality more visibile as a result of Jessie's female stem cells? Or, did my near-death experience and pre-existing traits shape my behaviour more prominently? Do my hormones differ? What kind of gene expressions have I inherited which wouldn't have existed were it not for the transplant? There are so many questions with endless possibilities, fascinating theories that deserve more attention. The eagle-eyed amongst you will notice I've made reference to such questioning on the cover of this book.

Mythology has always provided me with a different take on any situation I'm facing. It is in story that the deeper, unguarded parts of ourselves can be touched, making space for new perspectives. When revisiting the legend, I was stunned to read how Bellerophon, the male hero, kills the Chimera by lodging a lead-tipped spear inside the creature's throat. Her fiery breath melts the lead which blocks her airway and the Chimera dies by suffocation. This bares remarkable similarity to how my fate could have played out when my lungs were choked by bacterial pneumonia. Although I am a chimera, I see the pneumonia as the monster that needed to be defeated, rather than certain aspects of myself. Perhaps the echoes of this story will continue to be heard as I explore the trauma of forced ventilation, the subsequent fear of suffocation and all the subtle ways this continues to show up in my life.

While the mythical Chimera interests me as a genetic hybrid and describes curious parallels, it's not a creature I feel deeply connected to. There is another chimera I do feel a strong kinship with, however, one who is wrongfully – and quite literally – demonised.

Baphomet was first brought to public attention in 1856 via an image produced by Alphonse Louis Constant, working under the pseudonym of Eliphas Levi. In his book, *The Dogma and Ritual of High Magic*, Levi explained that the image was a representation of Pan and other archetypal horned-gods of fertility, pleasure, and hedonism. His image has been compared to the Devil card from the Tarot, which commonly shows a man and a woman chained to a block on which the horned one stands. Also wildly misunderstood, the Devil card represents our bond to the material world and shows up to signify when something is holding us back from being the best version of ourselves. Levi's depiction has since been twisted over time to become synonymous with a literal Devil, aka Satan, the Christian deification of pure evil.

Baphomet is clearly not the Devil, although that is what many people might see. Adopting this ancient god as an ally is not a pronouncement of extreme Satanism. I have not burnt any churches, nor am I now playing drums in a Scandinavian black metal outfit, but wouldn't that be an interesting twist to my tale? Rather than some child-eating monster, this divine chimera actually embodies pure, unashamed balance. As Julian Vayne and Nikki Wyrd so brilliantly set out in *The Book of Baphomet*, this archetypal deity is a unification of opposites, a god of all dualities; representing both male and female, life and death, human and animal, the light and the dark. Sounds like a great totem to have if you ask me.

For me, Baphomet is a reminder of the inherent paradox in the world; that humans are not all sweetness and light, good and evil deeds do exist and terrible things do happen, alongside the miraculous. Baphomet can help us embrace the darkness that we so frequently obscure. It shows death as a transformation, a natural and inevitable part of our lived experience. In many ways, it's an antidote to the modern condition of bypassing anything that brings up a fearful response; from the death of the individual to global concerns such as political and medical crises, the rise of extreme popularism, and environmental devastation.

Could Baphomet be an opportune call to self-empowerment, a gatekeeper of personal and global transformation? Its message is to take our heads from the sand and decide how we want to contribute to life today, not tomorrow. A valuable narrative, whether you choose to believe in such things as gods and deities or not.

Ω

Fire Made Flesh

When the old woman arrived home a few embers were still glowing. They spat and fussed as she opened the door to the burner, piling on a handful of kindling and a couple of fresh logs. She placed her bag down by the cabin door and unwrapped herself. The heat was precious now as outside the temperature had dropped. The wisdom of the flames would soon be called upon.

Her brew was ready, cooled to the perfect temperature to drink. Using a hand-carved ladle that had seen better days, she served herself a mug and took a few moments of rest. Reinvigorated, she cleared the floor in the centre of the living space, swept away the dust, long white hairs, and fragments of bark. From a cabinet on the far side of the room, she took a richly embroidered cloth, unfolded it, and laid it out. This was the ceremonial ground on which she would lay out the bones. This was the bedrock of her ritual.

She retrieved the skull of a female grey wolf from her altar and gathered together all she had collected that night. Then, as she had done so many times before, she pieced together the skeleton, sculpting it out precisely on the cloth, toe by toe, rib by rib, from the lumbar backbone to the tailbone. She finished with the pelvis and stood back to observe the result. She didn't need to check if all the bones were there, she could tell if one was missing simply by feel.

The fire was alive again now. Flames jostled, licking the glass as it grew hungry and demanded her attention. She took a cushion, opened the burner doors, and sat to greet it. Fire was an old ally of hers and over time she had learnt how to hear it speak. She knew how to ask of it and she knew how to give of herself in return.

As she stared into the flames, her voice returned. Low and deep at first, located in her belly. It began to move upwards with each breath, growing in volume. Her throat started to tingle as she opened up, allowing all sounds to flow freely. From guttural to animal, from a growl to a piercing whine, the old woman slowly stood and began to move her limbs. Eventually, a melody emerged from her throat; a song was being born. The fire was delighted and let her know, its sparks infused her song with a very specific ability; the power to revive a life.

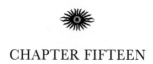

CHAPTER FIFTEEN

Prisoner

After my transplant I remained in the isolation room. I wasn't allowed out under any circumstances and only a handful of people actually ventured in. By the time I was permitted to return to the haematology ward, I'd spent the best part of a month living in that space.

Slowly but surely, my white blood cell count hinted at promising signs of growth. This meant that the bone marrow had, to some degree, assimilated into my bones and begun to make new cells. My count had to be above a certain threshold before they would consider my release, but we were all feeling the first flutters of elation at the idea of all this suffering finally drawing to an end.

In reality, things are rarely that smooth. As the days passed and my white cells bloomed, I tried to stay present with the process taking place inside me. I was easily exhausted by the smallest movements and was given daily transfusions of blood and platelets to keep me going. I dutifully practiced my visualisation technique in the shower, willing the great lake of white light far above me to flow down and spread throughout my body.

Years later I came to the conclusion that this practice can be understood as part of an innate self-healing mechanism. Rather laughable in conventional medicine terms no doubt, but I have a mind to trust my own sense of knowing on the matter. For this simple ritual made a noticeable difference to my wellbeing. Even so, I didn't tell anyone aside from my parents. Perhaps they thought I was going a little crazy from the stress of it all, I'm not sure. Either way, they made supportive sounds when I mentioned my experience but I noticed that they didn't enquire further. In a small epiphany, I realised that although I sought out their approval, I didn't need it. This autonomy spurred me on to develop an inner knowing of what felt right for me – a sense we generally call intuition. This kickstarted what has been a lifelong journey of trusting myself and trusting my body, listening to its wisdom, feeling into how it wants to move, noticing all the subtle ways I can detect what my needs are and respond appropriately.

As the white cell count kept on rising, my strength grew with it. I felt incrementally stronger; I had a little more energy, I was lighter on my feet and could move about the room without discomfort. I could even perform some very light stretching exercises. I realised how much better I felt simply by gently stretching my battered body, bending slowly over to the left, then the right, being careful not to snag my thick white Hickman line which dangled from my chest like a lonely plastic dreadlock.

We were now firmly into March, the month of my birth. Unlike many other young men around the country, celebrating their first steps over the threshold of adulthood by going out and getting legally drunk on weak lager, I'd spent my 18th birthday cooped up in an isolation room, hooked up to a drip. Tasha came over for a couple of precious hours, laden with gifts, soft kisses, and much-needed laughter. I inhaled her understated perfume as she slung her arm around me and nestled her head into my neck. We sat on the little sofa in my room sipping tea and eating chocolate biscuits. She grinned as my weak hands slowly unwrapped the birthday presents, taking delight in the way my face lit up.

My parents bought me a film camera, a nice little Canon, which I now wish I'd not been so keen to sell at the onset of digital photography. It gave me a window to hide behind, a way to step back and look at the world, recording for posterity whichever moments I chose to.

In the daytime, I would sit and chart the path of the world through the small rectangular window, positioned high on the far wall. By sitting in just the right spot I could follow a fluffy cumulonimbus as it lazily drifted by. The late winter sky shifted from light to dark without ever settling on one mood. With the actuality closer than ever, I allowed myself the luxury of imagining being out in the fresh air for real. No rules, no time limits. Freedom. How wild it would feel to have the warmth of the sun on my skin, or climb up a blustery Shropshire hill, my brand new baby hair blown about by the wind. I dreamed of the places we would go together, Tasha and I, kissing, laughing, having fun – living out a normal teenage existence.

The Earth continued to turn and the days all blurred into one. My routine was irritatingly simple. After getting up I'd take my long daily shower, graze at my breakfast tray and maybe listen to some music. In the afternoons I'd usually watch daytime TV. I became charmed by the old-school whodunnits; Peter Faulk as Colombo and Raymond Burr as the lawyer Perry Mason were my favourites. Their dated look and hammy plotlines carried me far away from my immediate situation.

A week or so after the transplant, as I began to get stronger and with the doctors making positive noises, my parents' daily visits were scaled down with one of them coming every other day. They needed time to tend to wider family issues and whatever else in their lives had been neglected in favour of caring for me. Typically, however, it was on one of the days I was alone that I underwent an attack of the worst pain I have ever experienced in my life, before or since.

I'd been dozing off to sleep, propped up by a mass of pillows. This way of sleeping, almost in a sitting position, was one I'd adopted ever since emerging from the depths of the Intensive Care Unit several months earlier. Following the rampaging pneumonia and MRSA, my chest had become my Achilles heel. Being upright allowed my lungs to drain more efficiently and my breathing to soften.

I'd noticed a couple of twinges around my right side earlier that day, but as I'd experienced all manner of bodily sensations since the early days of my treatment I didn't pay it too much attention. For a few hours, I slept. Sometime after midnight, I was awoken by a burning sharpness on the right side of my lower back. It felt like I'd been stabbed with a red-hot blade. The kind of pain that forces you to scream the word 'FUUUUUCK!' as loud as you can, while every muscle in your body convulses and tightens in an attempt to stem it. I writhed around groaning and swearing at the top of my voice. A night-duty nurse named Eva appeared at my bedside looking concerned.

'Oh you poor thing, Jody, can you tell me what's going on?' She mopped my brow.

'I'm… in so much… fucking pain,' I managed to say through clenched teeth. By now I was sweating profusely and the pain hadn't diminished in the slightest.

Eva added something to my IV. 'Keep breathing Jody, I've topped you up with some pain meds, they should kick in very soon.'

'Eva, could you phone my parents please?'

It was 1:30 am and they'd be sound asleep but I had to call them. She dialled the number and held the phone to my ear. It rang for a while and I pictured Dad rolling out of bed, eyes blurry from sleep, and Mum jolting into high-level worry mode about the manifestation of her worst fears. It was Dad who answered.

'Hello?'

'Dad, it's me, I need you. Everything hurts so much. Please come over.'

'Don't worry, Jode, I'm on my way.'

He must have driven like a demon and I must have dozed off, because all of a sudden he appeared in the room right next to me wearing full PPE.

He held my hand and kissed the top of my head lightly. I could see he was worried. We didn't know what was going on, we were both scared but he did his absolute best to be a rock for me to cling to.

Eva returned to check on me and dispatched another dose of painkillers. She'd spoken to a doctor who thought it could be a side-effect of the GVHD as my body adjusted to Jessie's new cells. Apparently, sometimes it could affect the liver.

Dad set up an armchair near my bed. After another hour of writhing in agony and heavy staccato breathing, I finally began to settle as the drugs kicked in. I drifted off into a delicate sleep with Dad dozing beside me, covered with a blanket, trying to get some rest himself.

In the desaturated light of the early morning, I awoke to see him still fast asleep in the chair. The pain had dulled into a numb ache. I felt completely exhausted. Soon after, Dad stirred as the nurses brought us in a simple breakfast. He was due at work that morning, so after making sure I was ok he showered and set off by 7:45 am. What an incredible man – the unconditional love he showed and the way he put himself to one side to care for me. I could barely speak my gratitude, it choked me so hard. After he'd gone, I cried streaky tears and felt strangely like the luckiest boy alive.

When the day finally arrived and I was allowed out of my little prison room, I felt elated. Utterly knackered, yet elated. The usually dense hospital air suddenly felt like the freshest of breezes. My entire body felt lighter. My soul still inhabited a frail and undernourished frame, moving slowly and delicately, but my mind was clearer than ever.

I was also calmer. I drew great strength from the fact I'd made it through the whole 'incarceration' time alive, with my greatest challenge now behind me. I had fresh bone marrow and my body was working feverishly to integrate it, generating a whole civilisation of healthy new cells. That was my hope, but of course, I didn't really know for sure. No-one did. This whole thing was now a waiting game, pure and simple. I had to remain patient, keep on doing my visualisations, keep asking my body to gently heal itself, keep making my silent prayers a morning mantra.

There would be some time now before the first bone marrow tests but all the signs were good. My blood count edged steadily towards healthfulness, which meant the doctors were happy to permit me a few days on the main ward. Once this count recovered to the required level I could leave hospital and return home to Bridgnorth.

On the day that I walked out of the haematology ward my confidence soared. Mum drove over to help me pack up and take me home. She was excited but trying not to let too much of it spill out. Prem had told us that the next few weeks were still critical and sent me home with a stapled-together booklet of printouts, documenting what I could and couldn't do, a whole range of medicines I was to take, and of course, a whole range of possible side-effects to be vigilant of.

Mum took notes and asked all the right questions while Prem's words bounced right off me. I glanced out of her office window and took in the view. The Edgbaston skyline spiralled out before me. It was as if the entire Universe both began and ended in this exact room, in that exact moment. Perhaps it did for me. I felt like I'd been given another chance, an opportunity to be reborn into a whole new beginning. I was seriously proud of myself for getting this far. 'Fucking good job, Jode. Every moment now shall be a gift,' I told myself. I didn't know quite how but I knew I'd strive to make my life count.

I'd been back home a little over a week. Mum and Dad were on the ball – helping me set up the drip stand for bags of saline, reminding me to keep my dressings clean and to be careful with the line still hanging out of my chest.

As somewhat of a water baby, I'd been fantasising about immersing myself in a hot bath for months. Taking a bath is one of life's simple pleasures. I'd made a silent promise to treat myself to one as soon as I was able and it was permitted. The guidelines said I mustn't fully submerge my Hickman line, so I gingerly ran the water to a level where I could safely lie down with just my upper chest sticking out, the rest of my body soaking in the glorious scented heat.

> **From:** Tash
> **Sent:** 5:11 pm
> Home then?! I'm so proud of you!!! T xxx

Despite being on a fairly restricted diet, Mum was able to whip up some of my favourite meals and I'd been excitedly rediscovering real food. Soon after I arrived home, we gathered around the dinner table to eat as a family. On the menu was Mum's Sunday roast, complete with all the trimmings. I'm sure everyone thinks their mum's roast is the best, but my mother really does know how to deliver the goods – 'It's all in the timing' – as she'd say.

The banter and familiar rhythms of our family interplay began to gently resurface now that we were reunited under one roof. There was a lightness to the occasion that had been very much absent since my diagnosis and everyone could feel the shift. Despite their good spirits, my parents looked tired, their lined faces betraying the stresses of the past six months. I remember looking around the table as a joke fluttered by, delighting in the laughter and silliness, taking in each of my siblings and feeling our invisible family connection deepening.

While I still needed plenty of rest I was able to see Tasha, which was always a buoyant moment. Sometimes she'd visit me or Dad would drive me over to hers. Every moment felt like a waking dream, as if I was still dosing myself with morphine. Riding high on a wave of post-hospital-release euphoria, I hadn't given GVHD much thought, other than dutifully knocking back the foul-tasting cyclosporin.

I was lying in bed at Tasha's house one blissful early morning, listening to the birdsong in the blue light, when she noticed a stippled red rash across my lower back. It became incredibly itchy and was accompanied by some twinges in my limbs and torso. We were both shocked. It was extremely deflating but I knew what had to happen. The next day it was back to the QE's outpatients clinic for an appointment with Dr. Mahendra who would be able to make a full assessment.

Yet another brief and tantalising taste of freedom. The cyclosporin had been working, doing its job to help my body cope with the influx of new cells, but evidently things had begun to get out of hand in cell-world. In the space between hope and expectation, a seed of doubt had sprouted. Thoughts of, 'Shit, maybe this thing won't actually work.'

The next few weeks were like this – back in the hospital for treatments, upping the cyclosporin dosage, then time at home to recuperate. After a couple of further flare-ups, the GVHD finally abated. It turned out I'd had it fairly easy. Many patients struggle long-term with it, and as I've mentioned, it can even be an outright killer.

As if awarding me some kind of twisted prize, life then decided to serve me up a full-on dose of shingles, the adult form of chickenpox. What typically manifests as a couple of days off school watching cartoons and a few itchy spots when you're young, can become excruciating, flu-like, and potentially deadly for the elderly or those with compromised immune systems.

Contracting shingles is shit. As if I didn't have enough to contend with; my body had barely gotten used to all the new cells flooding its organs and vascular systems, and now this. For fuck's sake. I was back on the ward for ten solid days, kept in a room for fear of being infectious, utterly wiped out, itching and scratching – against doctor's orders – under both arms and down the right side of my torso like an absolute madman, causing the rashes and swelling to get worse, often drawing blood and crying tears of sheer frustration.

As far as pain goes, it is right up there at No. 2 in my all-time top five. Here's some free advice: really don't get shingles. When we were kids Mum used to say, 'Better to have chicken pox now than get shingles when you're older.' She was right. Infection with the varicella-zoster virus as a child usually confers life-long immunity to it, but for those with compromised immune systems it can re-emerge as the nastier, more virulent shingles.

As you may have gathered by now, I wasn't going to give up easily. I fought on and worked through it. I endured as I'd endured before. I gritted my teeth. Nothing was going to defeat me at this point, with the light just about visible at the end of the tunnel. I dug deep and willed myself well – 'Just another hurdle to clear, Jode, you can do this.' My mind sparkled with determination while my body groaned and writhed in agony, blood-spotted sheets soaked with the sweat of another restless night.

Ω

Sounding Body

The old crone sang. Singing her heart out, she released any remaining sense of control and gave herself over entirely to the song. It wielded power. This she knew and trusted. Such power was an honour but she was not foolish enough to claim it as her own. This was a power inherited, handed down aeons ago, before there were Gods and before humans installed themselves as rulers of the Earth. Her melody twisted and spun in the warm air as it left her mouth, flirting with the wisps of woodsmoke escaping the burner. It arched up towards the dark moon.

Behind closed eyelids she saw flickering visions and spiralling geometry, life collapsing and reforming over and over again in an endless ancient dance. The image of a wolf sloped into her dreaming and suddenly she was face-to-face with its sparkling amber eyes. They stared back calmly, watching her.

The fire roared louder and the old woman moved faster, her limbs shaking. A chant emerged from deep within her lungs. Without stopping, she stooped to collect a rattle, shook it out with a chicka-chick, chicka-chick, chicka-chick, and began moving around the skeleton laid out on the cloth. Molecules moved and shifted in patterns of delight as she vibrated the air, calling in the animal, calling in new life. Her sense of self changed, as the soul that usually animated her body took a backseat, leaving a clear channel to the place of the dead and the not-yet-born. Now, spirit could enter.

Though she didn't notice at first, the bones had started to move. They quivered almost imperceptibly, resonating with her persistent rattle. The cabin opened up and the wolf blinked its amber eyes. The bones changed colour as life gushed in. Marrow thickened inside them. Flesh and blood vessels, muscles, and tendons appeared. They merged into the outline of a creature. The skin formed a pale greyish layer, knitting together the various organs and fascia that now covered the shape of this emergent body. She rattled harder, chanting a prayer to the fire, her intention crystal clear. The ritual was working. Hair started to form on the thickening skin, white and grey tufts became a pelt. A second layer grew and wrapped around the creature like a tightly woven shawl.

The wolf returned to her inner vision. The old woman called out her praise and gratitude to the animal. Her voice grew louder still, more determined. She began to wail with a raw ferocity. The cabin walls shuddered as she stamped out an insistent rhythm. Outside, the desert floor jumped in time with every beat. Whirling, spinning, consumed by ecstasy, finally she collapsed onto her knees, down beside the snapping flames.

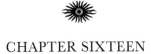

CHAPTER SIXTEEN

Moments of Clarity

Initially, I felt almost overwhelmingly delicate. I had been shown just how fast everything we hold dear can be pulled out from under us. I knew life was extremely precious. Let's be clear though, I was elated to be alive and for a time that was enough – to simply be living and breathing, taking each day at a time. We still had to go back to the QE once a week for an outpatients clinic with Prem, but my blood results kept improving and she seemed happy. I spent the rest of April recuperating, watching TV and eating when my appetite allowed. I still had my Hickman line in and I was still taking cyclosporin.

Within the space of six months, I'd spiralled rapidly towards death only to emerge anew. I was alive but fragile as a new-born, tired but holding the inner strength of a wolf cub, the softest layer of fur starting to grow. I survived an initiation I will never forget.

Beyond the thick of it, I stood in the clearing. As you might imagine, it changed everything. There was no map to help me understand what the hell had happened, nor how to move forward.

The excessive pain I experienced during the time of my illness – not to mention all the poking, prodding, pills, and puking – had the cumulative effect of bringing me into a deep awareness of my physical body. I had no choice but to face it as best I could. At times I fought against it, distracting myself – who wants to take that much shit? It isn't fucking fair. In time though, I learned to be patient with my ability to accept this reality. From this came bravery, I now knew I could deal with almost anything. It gave me balls – tiny hairless balls at that, but still, I grew courageous.

I had endless hours to lie on the bed feeling the sensations of my body. I'd listen to my heart thud a steady rhythm, pumping blood around the network of my veins and arteries. I'd flinch at the next muscular spasm and try to overcome the birth of every tingling itch. I'd endure the drip-bleep-drip of my IV machine, taking ownership of the ever-present flow of my breath whenever I could.

These functions whir away inside our bodies all the time, aiming to maintain the healthy balance that keeps us alive. If we are bold enough to turn away from distractions and spend some quiet time with ourselves, we may just notice them. After some time, perhaps we'd even feel a sense of peace as we learn to appreciate the biological miracle that we each are. It's similar to meditation, which usually involves the observation of the breath and the acceptance of all thoughts and sensations as tools to quiet our chattering minds.

I felt so tuned in to my body after I came out of the hospital. I listened when it spoke and tried to take decisions accordingly. I trusted in the messages my body fed back to me. My intuitive abilities were now amped to a whole new level. I had developed a degree of what you might call extra-sensory perception, but quickly realised that this way of being required regular practice to uphold in a fast-moving society. I needed to learn how to adjust the volume. I felt so alienated on my return and sought as much alone time as possible. The quiet solace of the countryside functioned like a recharging station for my mood and my sense of self. I'd really come to enjoy the simple feeling of being in my body with this newfound awareness.

Several months later, I discovered yoga. What started out as a sequence of muscle toning exercises, following Mum's Rosemary Connelly VHS tape, is now an integral part of my daily routine. Through numerous asanas (physical practices) and pranayama techniques (yogic breathing), I have learnt subtle ways of controlling my energy. Yoga has provided me with lifelong methods to help cultivate a relaxed body and a clearer state of mind.

Whilst I was mentally and emotionally coping, physically I was in a sorry state. The toll of the past few months was immediately obvious. Eighteen years of outdoor adventures, fresh air and good food had shaped me, but now all that was gone. I was frail and several stone lighter. I'd lost all the hair on my head and, to myself at least, resembled a gaunt being from a another planet. Like an olympic swimmer or a pornstar, my entire body was bald save for a few sparse gangster patches that had somehow clung on, refusing to leave. Having such smooth calves gave me low-level anxiety about baring my legs in public for years, although many of my female friends have expressed their envy.

In our family bathroom, directly opposite the bath, hung a large mirror covering one wall. I'd stand on the washed-out blue bathmat and gaze at the boy in the mirror. He was sad to look at, but there was a strength about him. I was actually still alive – sometimes I literally had to pinch myself. Staring at my nakedness, I'd look him right in the eye:

You did it, you fucking did it!

Yeah but look at me, I'm a shell, I'm a wreck. Tasha won't want to be with this half-man. I'm pathetic. I feel so alone.

Shut the fuck up dude! You fucking did it!

Tash reassured me that my appearance didn't matter to her, but the impact on my self-confidence had left a nasty bruise. I couldn't bring myself to accept her words, the change in me was too great. How could she see past this and still fancy me?

My mood was lifted by a trip to The Swan on Bridgnorth's High Street a few weeks later. A cold pint with my mates was a momentous occasion that I'd been looking forward to for months. As was tradition, Rob and I headed down town to meet the others. Walking in, a power-tripping young security guard took it upon himself to stride right up to my face, blocking my way.

'You're underage mate. I can't let you in without ID.'

Grim.

Unfortunately, I hadn't yet obtained any kind of official ID that didn't profess that my name was 'Jamie Whatts' and that I was actually twenty-one.

Hearing this, Rob turned on his heels, anger clearly rising on my behalf – the move of a true friend. He positioned himself squarely in front of the doorman, who was a good five years older as well as being rather well built.

'Don't be a dick, he's had fucking leukaemia! Besides, he's eighteen so you're gonna let him in.'

And so, he did. I savoured my first pint of beer in more than six months. Thanks, Rob, I'll never forget that, mate.

Returning to semi-normal activities was a big deal. I slowly sank back into the old routines, hanging out with friends around town. Nothing had really changed, everyone was still pretty much the same. Another year older, a little taller maybe and now sporting stubbly beards across the board. It also became clear they could handle their drink a great deal more than before. It was good to be back in a familiar groove and I enjoyed laughing along with the jokes, comforted by the inevitable banter. They even toasted my return to life, which was as heart-warming as it was embarrassing. For them at least, it appeared simple: Jody had been ill, MIA for the best part of a year and now he was back. No-one asked me too much about the specific events of my experience, except the inquisitive few who sidled up with their curiosity later in the night, away from the boozy hilarity.

Since my return from hospital, Jess and I saw a lot of each other around the house. Our relationship had inevitably shifted, and definitely for the better. Jessie, famous in our family for her long black eyelashes, found it hilarious that my own grew back looking almost identical to hers. She was also in admiration of my hair, a fluffy fuzz she'd nicknamed 'the baby soft'. My highly prized stubble had grown back very quickly, it was stronger, thicker, and darker than before.

Other fascinating things were starting to occur that appeared to suggest a degree of telepathic connection. I'd have a song running through my head all morning and Jess would happily waltz into the room singing it. We'd finish each other's sentences, often instinctively knowing what the other was feeling, both finding it ridiculous that we'd become so tuned into each other. I'm sure other siblings, twins, and close friends might report similar occurrences, but this was new for us.

In contemporary western society we are extremely quick to label metaphysical concepts as woo-woo or pseudo-science, yet it's clear that there is much about such events that fall outside the bounds of current scientific understanding. In 2018, however, there was a breakthrough. A Yale university study of a pair of conjoined twins, funded by the Defence Advanced Research Projects Agency (DARPA), led to what is being called 'proof of telepathy'. ABC News reported that despite having separate brains, the Canadian twins are able to communicate thoughts and see or feel each other's sensory input, even if their respective eyes are closed. Dr. Phillip Alveda, who conducted the brain imaging, is on record confirming that scientists 'now have a blueprint for communication from one brain to another.' Alveda goes further, suggesting that a device which enables human telepathy will be available within his lifetime: 'We can have telepathic communication, not just of vision, but of all our cognitive awareness. Imagine that situation. It's not a matter of if, it's a matter of when.'

★

As May arrived, promising warmth, I caught a nasty chest infection accompanied by a very high temperature. I was swiftly admitted to the newly built Teenage Cancer Trust Young Person's Unit at the QE, as the main haematology ward was full. It took several long hours to get my temperature down. Naturally, they were concerned about the infection developing into another potentially deadly case of pneumonia, given the weakness of my lungs. Had that happened, it would have been devastating at this delicate stage of my recovery. Copious amounts of antibiotics and vitamin-infused fluids finally stabilised me.

I remained on that bright and cosy little ward for the next three days, recovering my strength, playing games and hanging out with the other kid. After so many ups and downs, thankfully that was the last major hospitalisation I had to endure. As I recovered and my health grew steadily better, I took my first real steps on the long journey to rebuilding my life. Others were not so lucky.

You might remember Jane, the local lady who'd been battling lymphoma alongside me on Shrewsbury's haematology ward. We'd chatted in the outpatients department and the hospital car park many times, and had a mutual camaraderie. She'd been thrilled with my progress and so supportive. It saddened us all immensely to hear the cancer had aggressively returned, and this time they'd been unable to prevent Jane's death. My heart goes out to her family, Jane was a lovely person. With this news I felt luckier and more grateful than ever, especially for Jessie, as if I had somehow won a mysterious lottery.

In his classic work, *Rites and Symbols of Initiation: The Mysteries of Birth and Rebirth*, Mircea Eliade noted:

> *'It has often been said that one of the characteristics of the modern world is the disappearance of any meaningful rites of initiation.'* He continues, *'The majority of initiatory ordeals more or less clearly imply a ritual death followed by resurrection or a new birth. The central moment of every initiation is represented by the ceremony symbolizing the death of the novice and his return to the fellowship of the living. But he returns to life a new man, assuming another mode of being. Initiatory death signifies the end at once of childhood, ignorance, and the profane condition.'*

Rites of passage marking the evolution from child to adult, from dependency to self-sufficiency, are an essential aspect of tribal cultures which have been lost and forgotten along the journey to civilisation. As a species, we now find ourselves in the sobering position to reflect upon the damage that many generations of uninitiated humans have unwittingly caused. It is now up to us as individuals and communities to rediscover such frameworks, for ourselves, for our children, and for the planet.

Joseph Chilton Pearce was a brilliant and insightful American author, a highly regarded expert in child development, who devoted his life to exploring the incredible potential capacities held within each individual human being. Unusually for his time, Pearce blended cutting-edge science with holistic spirituality, understanding that to meet its future challenges effectively, humanity must tap into its innate ability for creative imagination – that space where the impossible becomes possible, where dreams can become reality.

Teenagers exist at such a precious stage of human development. They juggle youthful wildness with the fast-developing mind of an adult, navigating all the conditioning that growing up brings. In his groundbreaking book *From Magical Child to Magical Teen: A Guide to Adolescent Development*, Pearce coined the term 'post-biological development', referring to the stage that begins around the age of fifteen where identification with the brain has been withdrawn, and our identity as a being distinct from mind or body manifests and becomes stable. He states: 'Post-biological development opens us to creative power, a power of consciousness related to possibility rather than to what has already been created.' Pearce believed that once our outer models of the world are in place and our physical biology fully developed, a very natural process of opening to spirituality occurs which triggers the exploration of our unique individual potential. He believes living in such a way to be our birthright.

Many children begin the journey into life filled with innocence and wonder. As this is slowly flattened and moulded by parental and societal conditioning, the inherent magic and joy in simply being alive becomes forgotten. I acknowledge suffering and greed, selfishness and depravity exist in this world. I am in no way suggesting we bypass the storms of grief or anger that can arise in turbulent times. Being honest with ourselves and our emotions then finding safe ways to express them are important life skills.

As we grow through our teenage years, we are likely to move from idealising our life and how it might be, to feeling let down, unleashing a torrent of frustration, cynicism and rage as we convince ourselves that our dreams are futile and not worth chasing.

Despite this teen angst, some may germinate key seeds of inspiration at this stage. Perhaps they witness a performance of incredible artistic endeavour by master musicians, or watch, mouths open, as the circus rolls into town, masked clowns whooping their foolery while the ringmaster roams the stage. They may find embers of possibility nestled within their families, their circle of friends, or their wider communities. Moments of clarity, flashes of pure insight, and even great awakenings of consciousness can happen at any time, especially when you're least expecting it.

Such moments do not have to arrive in what we might consider a pleasant form either. Out from the ashes of horror, the fierce desire to understand and integrate can form. Perhaps one day it may even be transmuted. Even in the very hardest of times, there exist deep reserves of strength and resilience that we can draw upon. The willingness to fight for what is right and the desire to grow, learn and express ourselves can never be eradicated. Indeed, meeting challenges along the way can often end up making us even more determined to carve our own unique path.

Pearce observed that teenagers are pre-disposed to believe that 'something tremendous is supposed to happen, and supposed to happen right now.' He called this the *great expectation*. A feeling of longing, the heartache of constant anticipation. Following on from that come feelings of secret, hidden uniqueness – *if only the world knew who I really was and what I could do.*

Yet for a multitude of reasons, teens often have a difficult time finding the support they need at this crucial stage. Parental or guardian understanding can be stretched thin by the constant demands of adult life. Their ability to listen and empathise, remembering the days when they themselves were in the same shoes, can be so easily forgotten. Peer-groups are not always the most supportive of difference and individuality either – put simply, our friends can be fucking mean. This is why we so greatly need modern rites of passage.

Of course, any experience at any age can provide initiation into a more holistic and rewarding existence, but there is a reason why indigenous cultures often choose late adolescence as the time to hold specific rites of passage ceremonies. On the cusp of becoming an adult, the young person must attempt to honour their development thus far as a child, and then step forward on their own to prove their worth to the tribe and to the Earth. As Eliade describes, this unavoidably involves a death and rebirth process. The emergence into adulthood brings great responsibility as well as great freedom. Adolescence is a natural gateway where opportunity awaits those with the courage, resources, and support to take a leap. Imagine the possibilities for the world – not to mention our future as a species – if our teenagers were facilitated with access to their very own 'tremendous moment'. I think that is a world worth striving for.

Ω

Wolfboy

Slowly I opened my eyes. I was no longer falling through darkness. I was lying on a piece of material, laid out on a hard wooden floor. A hundred scents hit my nostrils at once and clamoured for attention: woodsmoke, burnt herbs, bare soil, blood. I heard the soft crackle of flames and somewhere beyond that, the flutter of mouse-feet. Everything sharpened in the dimly lit space.

Lifting my head, I caught sight of a plump older lady, swaddled in wool, sat quietly on a stool by the wood-stove. She fixed me with her wrinkled gaze and grinned, displaying a mouth full of yellowing teeth, tobacco on her breath. I looked down at where my arms should have been to see two large paws of mottled fur. My torso and legs were covered in this thick fur too. I began to panic – was I no longer human? What the hell was this place and who was this weird old woman?

I lurched to my feet, all four of my giant paws landing squarely on the floor. I circled shakily around the far side of the space, eyeing the crone, jumping back with a start as she moved. I opened my mouth to speak but all that came out was a low growl. She opened the door to reveal a blanket of pre-dawn mist, suspended below a gradient sky of pinkish-blue.

The opportunity to escape was clear and I made a bolt for it, leaping across the cloth and out through the wide-open door. With every sinew, muscle, and tendon suddenly working powerfully in unison, I raced forward into the sweet desert air. Running with four legs was exhilarating. The goldfish-bowl sky opened out above me, a ridge of mountains jutted off towards the westward horizon. With absolutely no idea where I was going, I ran towards the hills.

As the wolf-body moved faster I felt a shift start to occur. My limbs began to morph and change. A howling cry escaped my lungs. Confused, I glanced down and noticed my naked arms. Human arms with human skin. Then I was upright, my bipedal legs still working away, but no longer covered in fur. Naked as the day I was born, I leapt and laughed to myself, racing along a sandy trail with fire in my heart. Freedom. The sun peaked over the horizon to the east. Its first rays lightly kissed my skin. I was myself again.

CHAPTER SEVENTEEN

Adulting

Ever so slowly, life returned to a state of post-traumatic normality. My parents went back to work for the summer term, and with every passing week, I took another step forward. The family released a long collective exhale – as if they'd been holding their breath since the diagnosis.

I was scheduled to complete my final year of A-levels in September. All my mates would have finished their studies by then and moved on, while I'd be back sitting classes with the year below me, a handful of whom were already friends. Still, I knew I'd feel like the odd one out and wasn't entirely looking forward to it.

Tasha was preparing for her end-of-year exams so was frequently busy studying and completing coursework. Consequently, we weren't spending as much time together as I'd hoped and dreamed about.

I was still low on energy and couldn't manage much excitement. My days mostly consisted of sitting around the house watching daytime TV, reading, or playing on my Sony PlayStation, a gift from my parents to help me pass the time.

When Tash and I did hang out, we made a point to have fun. She knew I'd been through a nightmarish time and it was in her nature to make those around her smile, to radiate a certain carefree, happy-go-lucky sense about life. I relished spending time with her, almost to the point of obsession. She had stuck with me through my dramatic cancer journey and shown me all the love she had to give. I was dumbstruck with gratitude. Unfortunately for both of us, my damaged psyche had become attached to the idea of our relationship as a kind of human lifejacket. My quivering heart had taken her love and support as a sign of undying, lets-get-married-and-always-be-together commitment. Such teen delusions were compounded by the peak experience we had just been through. I began to see her not just as my girlfriend, but also my therapist and my therapy. I imagine she was well aware of the issues that could develop between us, she's a smart girl. For her, it was time to think seriously about a future beyond the bubble of our quaint little home town.

One May evening, Tash told me she was considering applying for a nursing degree at Bristol University, many hours drive from rural Shropshire. I was incensed by this news, my anger driven by the gripping fear that I might lose her. It threw me into a tailspin of panic; a key member of my post-trauma support team was thinking about quitting. In my inability to understand these dynamics objectively, I orchestrated an argument by pushing her to a position she didn't ask to be put in, a request for – and the secret expectation of – her undying love and affection. In my mind, she was the one being selfish. In reality, of course, she was moving forward naturally, entering a new phase of life, one that I was yet to reach.

Despite that friction, we had a glorious summer after her exams were finally over. We took sightseeing trips to ramshackle English market towns, got ourselves thoroughly lost on the wooded peaks of the Shropshire Hills, and canoodled our way around the riverside footpaths and cobbled streets of our pretty hometown.

We'd often hang out at her family's beautiful place in the country, making up for lost time by playing stoned board games through tremendous fits of giggles and feeding each other slices of pizza when the munchies hit. We were reacquainted with our nakedness, enjoying long-awaited sexual intimacy and talking late into the night. Through my rose-tinted glasses, I felt that things between us were even better than before my diagnosis. Her the extrovert, me the sensitive soul – complimenting each other perfectly.

Tash had a wide circle of friends and there were often many demands on her time. She'd made a decision to enjoy the summer together while making preparations for university, letting me down as gently as possible in the process. Not fully aware of the ramifications of this and beginning to feel threatened by the thought of her leaving, I responded by making unfair demands of my own that she was understandably unwilling to engage with. As a result, a silent distance began to sprout between us.

It had only been a few months since my transplant and my body was still adapting to the everyday world. Strictly speaking, I was not supposed to be drinking alcohol, eating fast food, or mingling in large crowded areas. Both my parents were worried about the idea when I suggested accompanying Tash and her friend Kath to V2000, our local large-scale music festival.

'Don't you think it's a bit too soon to be going to a festival, Jode?' Mum asked gently.

'No, I don't,' came my stubborn reply. 'The last bloods were the best yet.'

'Maybe we should phone Prem and check?'

'Fine, whatever,' I replied, my face sour. 'I didn't come this far just to sit around the house.'

I was desperate to show Tasha I was still a fun boyfriend, one worthy of her love and time. I hadn't yet realised the negative impact my deep-set emotional attachment to her was having. Prem had concerns too but said she wouldn't stop me from going. I promised to be vigilant when it came to food, germs, and substances of intoxication. My liver had taken a severe beating over the past year and booze really wouldn't help its recovery.

'See, she says it's ok.'

Mum looked a little defeated. Her and Dad exchanged quick glances.

'Ok Jode, if you promise to be careful and don't get carried away… You're not like all the other kids there, it's really important you remember that,' Dad said softly.

'I will, I will. I'll take all my pills and I know what foods to avoid.'

'Ok then. You make sure to call us if there are any problems. Is your phone charged?'

'I'll go and do it now.'

Dad dropped us off at the gates of Weston Park. Tash smiled sweetly and told him she'd keep me out of trouble. We trundled into the site with our backpacks, Tash carrying the tent. I'd been to the festival the previous year so I knew what to expect. It was late-August and Michael Fish had said it was going to be a scorcher. Mum had packed me a bottle of Boots Factor 50. Due to all the chemo, my skin would be more sensitive to sunburn and heat rash for up to a year. I had some fruit, a packet of crackers, tins of fish and baked beans. I was supposed to avoid anything with excess sugar or fat, deep-fried foods, and red meat. Chicken burgers it is then, I thought. A smile spread across my face as it dawned on me that I was here, alive and walking directly into one of my future visions, the scenes that had kept me going, a future that I wanted to live for.

Tash dropped the dusty green tent bag, her cheeks flushed. She was wearing a cute white t-shirt with the sleeves cut off and stonewash denim shorts. She nudged her sunglasses onto her head and turned to me.

'Here we are then, Jode! You made it this far.' She smiled and planted a kiss on my lips.

'I did, didn't I?' I couldn't quite place my emotions. I should have felt ecstatic but my shoulders were already weakening at the weight of my pack.

She took her phone out and began to fire off a quick text.

'I wonder where Kath is, we're meeting her at the Blue Camping Field.'

'Do you know how many of her mates are coming?'

'I think she said Tim, Rory, and Simon. I've met them a couple of times, they're posh rugby boys but they're good fun.'

'Right ok... I'm a bit worried about all the drinking, Tash. I'm only going to be able to do a pint or two at the most. I don't want to stop you having a laugh.'

She sat on her backpack and began to roll a spliff. 'Don't worry, you won't!' She grinned.

'I guess I just want you all to myself,' I squeezed her tanned shoulder.

'There'll be plenty of time for us, Jode, don't worry,' she assured me. She lit the joint and took a couple of drags. 'You good to get going?'

'Yeah, sure.'

I was full of nervous excitement to be back in the big wide world, doing things with the girl I loved, the girl who'd helped me get this far. We met up with the others and found a spot to pitch our tents amongst the multiple encampments now springing up across the hill. I'd met Kath before, she was a real hoot, cut from the same cloth as Tasha; a giver of no shits, bombastic in her desire to enjoy life. Her mates from boarding school seemed pleasant enough lads, they'd already cracked the beers out and were joking amongst themselves, but I could sense an air of entitled resentment growing inside me. Tash had slipped them a one-liner and they'd all fallen about as if it was the funniest thing ever uttered. Who were they to steal her attention, make her laugh? She was mine. Tash explained that I'd been in hospital recently, that there were some things I couldn't do. They nodded but didn't seem bothered. They were at a music festival to have fun, not to hear about my miraculous survival and months of struggle in a place somewhere between life and death.

We spent the first hours wandering around together in a loose gaggle, bouncing between the stages, tents, and the bars. I'd heard good things about a new group called Coldplay who were playing on the second stage mid-afternoon. We lay around in the warm sunshine – me slathered in suncream, Tash resting her head on my belly and leafing through the programme. I took sneaky sips from her cold pint of Weston's Cider. Chris Martin crooned sweetly about everything being yellow and all was right with the world.

That evening, as the sun began to set, I sensed myself apart from the group – the little boy ready for his bed. I'd had a cider, half a red bull, and several fake lemonades over the course of the day and I was growing tired. I pushed myself to catch a blissful performance by Morcheeba, which gave me a huge lift, just enough energy to carry me into the night.

Tash was doing her best to enjoy herself. She was done with the trappings of school for a while, her life was unspooling ahead of her; of course she wanted to blow off some steam, she deserved it. In my tiredness, in my selfishness, I felt she wasn't giving me her full attention and quietly began to resent her, as well as the rest of the group for pulling her away. The seeds of my first post-treatment meltdown were duly planted. As far as I was concerned, no-one else deserved to invade our quality time. She was my girlfriend, my saviour, my angel. I coveted her. I needed her. Fuck the rest of them, they hadn't just been through what we'd been through.

After the main stage closed around 11 pm, the yawning kicked in. My legs ached from all the walking and I felt myself needing the warmth of my sleeping bag. The others were keen to continue their evening and had drifted into disparate pairings. The vast blue peaks of the club tent boomed out a thud-thud-thud to the gurning young faces, as the rest of the site slowly deployed its attendees back to their flimsy tents.

'Shall we go back, Tash? I'm knackered,' I said.

She seemed unsure, torn between her duty to look after me and her desire to go out and party with her friends.

'Kath, what are you lot doing now?'

'We're going to go to the club tent I think. Goldie's on at half-one.'

'Hmm, sounds good.'

'Come back with me…' I whispered, doing my best hangdog expression.

She looked at me, I could see her thinking.

'Thanks mate, but I'm going to head back with this one, have a good one!'

As she settled into her sleeping bag, I reached out for a cuddle and we fell asleep with our heads almost touching, both in our separate bags. Just as the residual chatter had died down, someone started the time-honoured, British festival tradition of shouting 'Bollocks!' at the top of their voice. This was repeated by others nearby, passed along from tent to tent in weird and wonderful ways until it had snaked its way across the field like a lairy virus.

The next morning I stretched out as my consciousness returned to the waking realm. The tent was humid and I was desperate for a piss. Tash was still sound asleep when I returned so I sat outside on a blanket, made a cup of tea, and lit the last remnants of her bedtime spliff. I shouldn't really have been smoking but I found cannabis really helped take the edge off my yo-yo-ing emotions. I needed to balance myself somehow to get through it.

The second day went similarly to the first. My underlying resentment hadn't shifted, it coloured the whole day. I looked around at the thronging crowd of strangers, intent on getting wasted, laughing, and joking. I felt disgusted. Fuck them. I began to seethe. Tash could tell something was up.

'You ok, Jode? Have a sip of this.' She offered me her plastic pint cup.

'No, I'm fine. I shouldn't be drinking. Drinking is fucking stupid.'

'Oh, so I'm stupid am I?'

'No, no, not you. I mean… getting wasted is stupid. Don't these people understand how frail their bodies are?'

'I guess they don't want to think about that right now.'

'Fucking idiots.'

'Hey, hey. Calm down, Mr Angry.'

'I'm going back to the tent, Tash, I need to lie down.'

'You sure?'

'Yes, very.'

'Ok, well I'll come back and check on you in a bit, alright?'

'Ok,' I answered. I gave her a firm kiss, gathered my bag, and made my way back, cheeks stinging.

I lay in the tent, stewing in my emotions, trying to nap. At some point, I must have drifted off because I was woken by the zipper. The sun was starting to hang low. Tash's head poked through the flap, concerned.

'Do you feel like coming back out, Jode? Moby is playing tonight, it should be a good one. We just came back to stock up.'

Just looking at her stung my eyes with tears.

'No, no. I can't.'

She clambered inside and put her arms around me. 'What's up?'

'This is bullshit, Tash, all these people getting wrecked. For what? Can't we just stay here, you and me?'

'If people want to have fun that's their business, not yours,' she prickled. 'I'm having a good time and I'm going to head out with the others tonight. Why don't you come out, you might feel better?'

'No. I won't,' I replied. I forced out more tears to amplify the intended effect. 'I want to stay here with you. Why can't we do that?' I asked. I wanted her to see me break. I wanted her to stay here and fix me.

'I'm not doing that, Jode, you're being selfish now. By all means, stay here if you want but I'm going out.' She grabbed a hoodie and a fresh pack of cigarettes and backed out of the tent.

'I'll be back later, alright? Text me if you change your mind...'

I heard her tell the rest of them that I wasn't coming out. A couple of people asked if I was ok. She replied that I wasn't feeling great. As they left for the evening, I sat on my heels, rocking back and forth, the sleeping bag pulled up under my armpits. One day at the festival had been manageable, two was too much. I felt weak and powerless, unable to fit into normality like everyone else, and hating them for it. Hating the crowds, hating this group of people. The way I saw it, Tasha had abandoned me and that was what hurt the most. I thought about calling my parents and asking them to collect me, but instead, I spent a couple of hours sobbing into my pillow until finally falling asleep.

It happens sometimes when we're deep into destructive or selfish behaviour: an observational awareness can rise like a drone above and behind us. This observer recognises we are being complete idiots in the moment, yet the part of us invested in the drama can find it nigh on impossible to snap out of it, apologise and ask for forgiveness. I wanted the argument. I wanted her to see me broken and in need so she could come running to fix me, to hold me, and keep me safe. And goddammit if she wasn't going to fall for it. She was too smart to play into my victim games. I was left as the successful architect of my own breakdown, refusing to look at the reasons why I had facilitated such a situation – the wounded fool in a sweaty blue tent in the middle of thousands of others just like it, whilst outside everyone else was having the time of their young lives.

The next morning, I managed an apology to the group, playing the illness card. I resolved to try and enjoy the last day of the festival but knew I'd driven an uncomfortable wedge between us. It killed me to acknowledge it and so I made an effort to be as normal as possible. Still, something had changed. Later, when we were alone, I apologised profusely to Tash for the way I'd behaved the previous night. She brushed it off, but I could tell that now she saw me through different eyes.

I returned to school as Autumn fell once more. Almost a year on from my diagnosis, I re-joined my old teachers for English, Geography, and IT, this time with the familiar faces of the kids in the year below who all treated me kindly and with sympathy. They were a good bunch and understood my situation.

Bristol University had accepted Tasha's application for a nursing degree but she'd decided to defer her place until 2001, taking a gap year with the aim of going travelling. I appreciated her support as I re-adjusted into the rhythms of normality, although we argued more and more. The unspoken tension around her going away and my refusal to accept our inevitable breakup was forefront whenever we spent time together. It was a matter of when, not if, yet despite the fattening dossier of evidence, I managed to convince myself that it simply wouldn't happen. This dreamer could imagine anything and dream it into a potential reality, especially the alluring story that Tasha would choose to stay with me after all. It was a lifeline I clung to hopelessly.

From: Tash
Sent: 3:02 pm
We need to talk, come to The Bell at 6pm T xx

Shortly after our last Christmas together as I grew clingier, she made her final decision. I imagine everyone saw it coming, except me, who'd refused to. Even though part of me knew exactly what she meant by *we need to talk*, hearing her say the actual words and feeling the real-time death of our romance destroyed me. I was deeply attached to her and the idea of our relationship being a teen-movie kind of love, but that wasn't real or even remotely attainable; it was pure fantasy. When we broke up, that dream was shattered and my heart cracked open. I was an inconsolable mess for days. I cocooned myself in my bedroom, barely eating, sobbing puffy-eyed into my t-shirt. I couldn't comprehend how life could go on without her.

I'd built this girl up into something more-than-human, a kind of angelic deity who'd been with me through one of the most challenging experiences it is possible for someone to have. *Of course* I wanted her to stay with me. At eighteen years old I hadn't yet gained the emotional intelligence necessary to allow her to make her own decisions and to respect that she needed to make her life the priority. I was irrational and for a while, my sense of perspective stopped right in front of my eyes. She'd fucked me over and that was it. Yet I found it impossible to hate her for it for more than a few seconds at a time. I was still hopelessly in love, or so I thought. There followed a dramatic love-hate spiral of anguish and resentment, of needless suffering as I told myself that no-one else could ever live up to her. I imprinted the idea that after her there was no point considering being close to another girl. As Sinead sang – *nothing compares to you.* She knew what I was feeling. Nobody would ever understand me the way Tash did. Why should I even bother trying?

My role as the classical hero had begun to break apart. The myth was starting to fail me. Fresh out of my cancerous initiation, I was convinced that life had lifted me up only to let me down. I'd overcome the tremendous threat of death but I hadn't got the girl, hadn't come home to the village in the kind of glory I'd so often envisaged. I was alive, yes, but battle-scarred and deeply wounded, wrestling with a cloying sense of detachment to other people and the day-to-day rhythms of reality. After getting so far, losing Tasha felt like an excessively cruel blow to my fragile teenage ego. I didn't possess the maturity to make sense of it.

One thing I had learnt from my cancer experience though, was how to compartmentalise. After a couple of weeks of moping around the house and making everyone feel sorry for me, I picked myself up, buried my grief at this painful loss, and turned my focus to the remainder of my studies. I began to enjoy life again; returning to play music with friends, getting high, studying hard. I left Bridgnorth Endowed School with three B grades at A-level in English Language, Geography, and IT. I applied for a BSc Multimedia Computing degree at De Montfort University in Leicester and tried to move forward, all the while missing her terribly, all the time feeling as if I was living in a peculiar bubble that no other could ever truly enter.

The internalised belief that *I would never find another like her* would turn out to be one of the most life-limiting for me, especially where sex and love were concerned. I tried to convince myself that someday, it could be decades away, Tasha and I would be reunited. In truth, I wasn't ready to open up to anyone else. I had to get to know Jody again. To better understand what I'd been through and how it had forever changed me, I needed time on my own.

While my friends were out living the hedonism of normal university life, I was turning inward to spirituality and psychedelics, devouring books on psychology and lucid dreaming. Tasha had been the one thing keeping me attached to my adolescence. The ending of our relationship was another small death that I was forced to confront whilst in a very vulnerable state. It left me with a deep fear of rejection and a strong desire to protect myself against any further heartache. Consequently, I held any possibility of intimacy at arm's length in those unfolding years. As a freshly minted adult, opening up to the kind of love that would no doubt be a catalyst for my own emotional and psychological healing was terrifying. It would have to wait. Whilst this was a necessary period of integration that provided valuable space for self-understanding, I let it go on far longer than was healthy.

Tash achieved what she set out to do, completing her studies in Bristol and qualifying as a paediatric nurse. She worked in a local hospital for a time before finding it all too restrictive. I have no doubt she touched plenty of lives. Whilst we are in touch via texts and email, we've not seen each other in person now for a decade or more. I am very happy to tell you, however, that she has read this book and given it her full approval. I hope to deliver Tasha's copy in person, after all, without her I don't know if I'd still be here to tell the tale.

For the six months following discharge, I had weekly checkups at the QE to monitor my blood counts, kidney and liver function. This included checking my bone marrow with a good old-fashioned lumbar puncture every two weeks. My fondness for that sweet post-midazolam feeling was still intact, so I wasn't particularly bothered about going in for the procedure. By now I knew it well. After a few of these, Mum's patience began to wear a little thin. Each time she'd have to deal with navigating her partially-high son, bent over and wobbling, down to the car park with him intent on hitting up the hospital shop for an alluring pack of Skittles, babbling about his tripped-out visions like a sun-baked preacher, then promptly falling asleep in the car on the way home, remembering almost nothing the following day.

I was on a very strict diet and could only introduce normal

teenage activities as I felt ready for them, and only then with the prior agreement of Prem and her team. She advised taking penicillin for at least the first six months and then at any sign of illness for the entire rest of my life. It was the only recommendation she'd made that I had a strong negative reaction to. To me, that approach seemed to be more damaging than helpful long-term, so I agreed to take it for half a year or so and then stopped as my health returned.

Prem told me that as my recovery progressed and my blood counts remained stable, the outpatient visits would be reduced to every fortnight and then once a month. Eventually, this worked its way down to just once a year. My final checkup was around the tenth anniversary of my transplant in 2010. Dr. Tim Corbett, haematology consultant at the University of Sussex Hospital in Brighton, where I was living at the time, took one look at my consistently stable blood count and said he didn't need to see me anymore. As I write, it is the year 2021 and I've been free of cancer for over two decades. My sister's bones and their miraculous pink goo live on inside me.

These days, I am well and healthy. People tell me I look young for my age. I have even been known to get ID checked when buying a bottle of wine from time to time, which always makes my day as I near forty years of age. I figure I must be doing something right. I have all my own teeth with no fillings and rarely catch so much as a cold. I'd be lying if I said I never thought about the leukaemia returning though, or if I told you I now lived a happy-go-lucky, fear-free existence. Those thoughts do sneak their way in, but I know my body and I listen to it deeply. When it speaks, I trust its messages.

On occasion, encouraged by the dampness of a British winter, I suffer allergic asthma attacks. My upper chest tightens and it is difficult to take a full breath. It's also triggered by dust or mould. At those times, I can feel my thoughts begin to sway precariously towards the cliff of anxiety. They even have the power to tip me into the ocean of full panic. Over the years, I've learned many ways of managing my feelings and thoughts, working directly to calm my nervous system. Some of my favourites include yogic breathing, qi gong, cannabis, meditation, and simply sitting with my back resting against the trunk of a grand old tree.

Any issues with my breathing send me right back to the ICU. I'm immediately back in the CPAP mask, experiencing the violence of forced ventilation. Back on the bed, drifting between worlds, teleporting myself into various elaborate and hyperreal morphine dreams, my frail body fighting to survive and those around me unsure if I would make it through that long, tense night.

While the trauma of this experience can still feed any latent anxiety I might feel in the present, I am forever grateful to be bolstered by a sense of what I can only describe as a *sacred warrior* spirit. Ever since my experience, it has remained deep inside me, right in the centre of my chest. It teaches that whatever situations and circumstances life has in store for me, I know beyond any shadow of a doubt that I can face them. That courage is nothing less than a blessed gift for which I give thanks to my leukaemia and all its associated trauma. For even that which may have whisked my young life away, also held within it the possibility of becoming my greatest teacher.

Epilogue

When the hero returns from his brave quest and the adversary has been overcome – in my case the apparent defeat of cancer – what then? It's convenient for certain fairytales to end it there: 'They survived, they came home victorious – The End.' But that is part of a much broader story. To follow the framework of the myth, I was to return to ordinary life with an elixir – a distillation of the very essence of the journey, something to share with my community. Without that, who was I? Apparently not much of a hero.

I definitely needed counselling in those early years post-treatment, but I was too physically and emotionally spent to consider it myself. I recall firmly rebuking my parents' gentle suggestions of talking to a professional. Fear told me personal therapy was something broken people did, while there I was all freshly fixed-up and reborn. I didn't want to direct my attention to those long months of upheaval, I just wanted to move forwards.

Little did I know that upon my return from this descent, this *katabasis*, I would be deposited right at the beginning of another cycle of transformation. Another turning of the wheel of self-understanding. It would take almost ten years, spanning the majority of my twenties, to move through the next stage.

How much do myths shape our lives? This vital question should be explored in every school classroom throughout the world. In my case, the hero myth was extremely well executed during my time in the hospital. It's important to respect the impact of the other characters in this story, to remember that I also owe my life to the people around me: the doctors and nurses, the consultants and other hospital staff, my family and Tasha, those friends and relatives who prayed for me, sent me mixtapes, and held me in their thoughts, the strangers who donated blood, and those who ground up my pills. They all contributed to my healing.

The myth gave me a roadmap for how to act and what to feel, especially in those initial stages. By engaging with the archetype in the short-term, I truly believe my chances of survival were greatly increased. During the process, my enemy became not death itself, but its potential facilitator, my renegade cancer cells. Yet what are the longer-term consequences – does the myth still work after it has been lived out?

Being cast as the hero came with serious baggage. Because I survived, against all the odds with a prognosis of just two weeks, I returned lugging a heavy sack of obligations. Firstly, I felt a responsibility to my family, who had made great sacrifices so they could support me through it all. Now I'd need to make them extra proud, to show them it was all worth it. I also felt an obligation to life itself for giving me a second chance to be alive and kicking on this blue planet.

All this weight brought recurrent waves of guilt. I shouldn't be messing around by going off to university. I should be getting out on the road, fundraising for cancer charities, doing sponsored walks and motivational speaking tours, espousing to the public how to live for today, and telling tales of how I slayed the cancer demon and thus postponed my appointment with death. These thoughts flew around my young mind and put immense pressure on me to achieve something astounding. To be an inspiration. To make my second chance really count. To be worthy.

How on earth is an emotionally immature eighteen-year-old with an underlying case of PTSD expected to cope with such a daunting task? I could either succumb to the burden of living up to this most incredible victory or try my best to live each day in defiance of survivor's guilt.

Being the one at the centre of the journey, I was a focal point for love and attention. Specialness was projected onto me consistently. In our society, we have a strange tendency to make cancer patients into celebrities, as if suffering itself is something to be celebrated.

I stumbled out of my teenage years with the idea kicking around my head that maybe I was special. Maybe I had been granted this rebirth by some kind of higher power via the medium of Jessie's bone marrow. Great things were destined to come my way. For a while, I was happy to go along with that narrative, but I couldn't be sure if it was actually true. Who doesn't want to feel special? It felt good to be granted a platform. It felt good to tell my story, watch the person's expression shift and feel their intrigue and admiration.

The more time I spent in the real world, with all its unfairness and adult responsibilities, the more the divergence between my mythic and practical realities became palpable. I had embodied the hero archetype to survive – in mythic terms I was *the hero who vanquished death*. Where was my special status to carry me next in life? Which kingdoms would I rule over and where were my crowds of fawning acolytes? Surely that was the least I deserved? Almost unavoidably, I carried an exaggerated sense of my own importance.

The word 'special' unsettles me. It creates a duality – those who are and those who are not. We have been dealing with the aftermath of people marked as special for centuries. In organised religion, priests are special as they are the chosen servants of God. There exists a hierarchy. The congregation are simply the followers who must do what they are told and who cannot be trusted to think for themselves. Similarly, our ruling classes and political leaders appear happy to designate themselves superior to the electorate by virtue of their schooling, bloodline, or social status. As if somehow only they know best.

The hero myth appears often within adolescence. During that critical stage of individuation when a young person is developing their ego, their sense of who they are in relation to the world around them, they can be strong-willed and impassioned – on a quest to find themselves. Of course, this quest never truly ends, but as obstacles are overcome the teens mature into adults, willing and able to share the elixir with their communities.

Should they remain invested in the battle, unable to grow beyond it, the hero myth can become destructive. This can manifest in a variety of ways, but we see it most in those who seek power and status, who are deeply attached to selfish outcomes. Such discontented individuals get stuck in dominant, overtly masculine attributes – all fight and no flow, you might say. In the book, *The Journey of Soul Initiation*, visionary teacher Bill Plotkin explores what becomes of a culture unconcerned by the resulting lack of 'true adults'. Plotkin would term them 'psychological adolescents' – people who covet their rewards and cover their ears to the call for self-reflection, who age without maturing.

Growing into a balanced adult requires the receptive, yielding qualities of the feminine alongside the direct drive of the masculine. Whilst I believe that the realisation of the individual and their gifts is key to the evolution of our species, it is quite clear that our over-reliance on selfish, human-centric thinking has spiralled out of control, as those in power refuse to see the irreversible damage being done to the planet in the name of progress.

Thankfully, I was brought back down to earth from the transcendent tendencies of my twenties by my close friends. The ability to laugh at myself helped deconstruct the heroic sense of specialness I had been feeling. Humility taught me that people may label you with all the terms they wish to, it doesn't really matter. What does matter is the way their words land in you. This requires a certain degree of maturity. Placing people in a hierarchy because of their personal abilities and circumstances can lead to false icons and jealousy, as celebrity culture ably demonstrates.

My cancer experience in no way makes me any better than anyone else. I was treated as special by everyone around me and for a while that was the way it had to be. It was the hardest time of my life. I barely got through it. It tore me apart, launched me into wondrous and terrifying changes of consciousness, all on the cusp of adulthood. Not exactly your average eighteen-year-old's night out with the lads. It broke me, changed me, and inspired me in ways others will never be able to fully understand. Did survival set me on course for a unique destiny? It certainly shaped me into the man I am today and inspired the path I have followed thus far. To make it through, I had to become the hero but that does not mean I am forever the chosen one. The myth broke down as I realised the impossibility of defying death.

Is it our fear of death that lies at the root of many of our deepest fears? I have often wondered this. For the majority of my childhood, I didn't have much involvement with death. As a kid I don't know if the thought of my mortality even entered my head; it was such a distant concept, something that mostly happens to old people, nothing to worry about right now. Moving from this position of vague awareness to the sharp reality of facing my own demise, and later witnessing others die in hospital, was a radical perspective shift. I was forced to accept my dying.

That pivotal year led to many unfolding deaths. The obliteration of my bone marrow before the transplant emptied my bones of their lifeblood. As the adolescent became an adult, my child self began to die, beliefs and opinions forming independent of parental approval. The innocent youth who walked into that isolation room unsure if he was going to return emerged reborn – kickstarting an awakening of consciousness. A few months later, the death of my relationship with Tasha released us both into the freedoms of adulthood.

Thoughts of dying didn't phase me for years afterwards. Not much did if I'm honest. These days, I have my moments – especially when the part of me that would rather not have to think about all that stuff rears its head. Even after such an acute near-death experience, I still need to remind myself that it is not something to fear. We shall all one day die, our bodies returning to dust in the ground, each fulfilling our role in the endless natural cycle. There is immense beauty in death and making our peace with it is essential to living a life in which we are fully alive. Remembering this as we go about our daily business can infuse every breath, every action and decision with a sense of clarity that is hard to come by through other means. I regard it as perhaps the ultimate spiritual teaching.

The understanding I have come to is that there is no enemy, and therefore nothing to fear. Life leads us all to a transition point. Death is not an ending but a beginning – cycles within cycles. The inevitability of our dying is a reality we must all come to terms with. There is no avoiding it. I believe that how a society faces up to death is a sign of its overall health. Long-standing cultural fear in the West tells us it is nigh-impossible to experience a good death. Death and dying are still very much taboo subjects, loaded with negativity. We are raised to believe that death is something far-off and scary, an unknowable event we should avoid thinking about until it happens. This is an act of pure repression. Mentally preparing ourselves for dying and cultivating an ongoing acceptance of our physical impermanence is time well spent.

In the Prologue, you may recall I mentioned the potential of using spiritual alchemy as a framework for personal transformation. I consider the writing of this book to be a form of alchemy in itself; gradually turning leaden pain into the gold of lasting good health, the embrace of my gifts, and the drive to make a positive impact on my own small corner of the world.

In Eliphas Levi's illustration of the deity Baphomet, the words *Solve et Coagula* are tattooed on its forearms. This translates as *Solution and Coagulation* and describes quintessential alchemical procedures. In solution, something is broken down into its smallest components or base elements. Throughout several stages, it is cleansed of any impurities and finally reassembled into a more useful or valuable substance – this is coagulation. Together they describe a process I have undergone many times now; in the hospital, in pushing myself to grow past my old stories, in searching for answers, and in writing this all down here for you to read.

You have been reading about an experience that came incredibly close to killing me. It took years of self-inquiry, deep dives into yoga, shamanism, and a fairly consistent meditation practice to even scratch the surface of what needed integrating. Over the years, however, one thing became abundantly clear: my illness was a kind of shamanic sickness – an initiation through pain and altered states of consciousness into alternative perspectives on the nature of life and death. Discovering the mind-body connection through my dreaming revealed the existence of vast archetypal realms.

What did this all mean? How was I supposed to apply these gifts of perception I had unlocked? I had no framework for understanding, so I became an apprentice. Initially, I followed the path of my culture and read books, watched documentaries, and attended workshops. Later, I got serious and began to work longer-term with genuine teachers who I trusted. More importantly, I was able to open my eyes and see the world through the lens of animism, vital and alive, buzzing with information. To my initial surprise, I found that when approached in this way *the world looked back*. It was open to my communication. It spoke to me through dreams and symbols, synchronicities, and impossible-to-ignore gut feelings. These communications came easily and naturally, as if I had tuned into a rare radio station that was usually hidden amongst the static.

As cultural mythologist Michael Meade describes in his book, *The Genius Myth*, every human being is birthed into the world with their own unique kind of genius fully intact. In this sense, genius is born, not made. Thinking of genius as an aspect of the soul means we arrive on the Earth with our particular gifts and abilities stored away inside us, ready to unfurl. Outside events will undoubtedly influence the path we choose, but remembering that we hold the keys from the very start is deeply empowering.

Twenty years on, I have come to see my illness as nothing less than a precious gift. No longer my enemy, but my teacher. This apparent contradiction of the myth was puzzling at first, yet the more I thought about it, the more it felt true. When I started to talk about this with friends and family it took them a while to grasp what I was saying. How could I possibly feel gratitude for my cancer? After all I went through, nearly dying, all the stress that put on those around me, how on earth could I consider it to be a *good thing*?

Despite weighing myself down with the worries and expectations of survival, it turns out my only real obligation was to stand knee-deep in the compost of my life, digging, weeding, and preparing the soil, so that I may finally share my experience and sow the seeds of the next phase. Only with proper reflection could I communicate what really went on. That is the path I have been guided along, one of attempting to find the gold hidden within this story. After writing was complete, I realised something: this book is my elixir.

How then will this story be transmuted? What is the gold I have alchemised? Wisdom is personal and timely; one person's diamond is another's roughly-hewn pebble. I hope that in reading this book there might have been a scene, a moment, an idea, or an emotion that resonated with you. Perhaps it caused you to question a belief, to more deeply explore a passion you have or a project you want to birth, or simply to open your heart again and give yourself a little more kindness. Perhaps you were moved to donate blood and stem cells, or maybe you were comforted by reading about someone who has been where you are. If the answer to any of those scenarios is yes then I can count this work a success.

On a personal level, the act of writing this story down has the effect of transforming it into something I can freely release. Whilst the events of that time are vital chapters in my unfolding personal mythos, ones which I honour as the greatest challenges of my life thus far, they have the potential to become shackles around my ankles, weighty scapegoats for all my unresolved issues. The resolution comes through an ever-evolving awareness, spiralling out to see the bigger picture, neither disowning them nor remaining defiantly attached. Like a former lover who will forever have a place in our hearts, but with the passage of time and the living of separate lives no longer exerts any influence over us, our present relationships, or our future decisions. We may kiss those magical memories lightly, honouring their role in the story of our life, and then simply leave them be.

Acknowledgements

Firstly, I must thank all the incredible doctors, nurses, hospital staff, and caregivers of the Royal Shrewsbury Hospital NHS Trust and the Queen Elizabeth Hospital, Birmingham circa 1999-2000, especially Haematology Consultants Dr. Nigel O'Connor – now retired – and Dr. Prem Mahendra. My deep gratitude goes out to the indomitable Haematology Nurses in those first months of my treatment – Luanne, Emma, Mary, Helen, and all the golden-hearted angels who helped carry me through.

I give thanks for my immediate family – Mum, Dad, Jemma, Jessie, and Josh – for being the ultimate rocks of love and support in all I do, even the really weird shit. I literally would not be here without you. Not forgetting the four-leggeds: Kelly, Mac, Meg, and Flo. To all my extended family; Uncles, Aunties, Grandparents, Cousins, and Godparents who helped me get this far, I love you all.

To the luminous girl who stole my young heart, who had no idea what she was getting herself into, but stuck with it all the way – Tasha, you got me through.

There are also people without whom this book would have been a pale imitation of its finished form. I thank those who helped me shape and refine it into the artefact you see before you. A hug, a firm handshake, and a complimentary bacon sandwich to maestro Ian Marchant – celebrated author, radio personality, creative writing tutor, and Presteigne legend. Deep thanks to you, sir, for seeing the potential in my work and encouraging me to make it better, bolder, and more daring.

Thanks also to Catherine MacCoun, author and alchemist, who reviewed an early draft and raised some big questions around the mythology that went on to inform the scope of the final book. If you're interested in alchemy as a spiritual practice, her book On Becoming An Alchemist (Shambala, 2017) comes highly recommended.

Deep thanks to Wendell Berry – yes *the* Wendell Berry – who not only replied to my letter from across the big sea in Kentucky, but was also kind enough to give me permission to use his stunning poem *To Know The Dark* as the epigraph to Part One.

High praise to all the skilled and friendly independent helpers I employed through the Fiverr website: Beta readers @Sarahmaew, @Monicam1001, and @Catherinbooks, editing by @Thpeditingservc, and invaluable proof-reading by @Katieevelynm.

Thanks to all those friends who have supported me over the years with their time, kindness, and laughter – from Bridgnorth to Brighton, from St. Leonards to Presteigne, and everywhere in-between. Especially you persistent ones who have politely inquired about my progress on this project in recent years. It all helped me keep going.

A special mention must go to Mark Golding, to whom I give credit for suggesting the title of this book.

Thanks to Jayne Worthington for the amazing cover photography, Russell Lewis for the jazzy promo shots, Marta Zubieta for the wonderful illustration, and Rural Media for the crowdfunder video. Big thanks to the patient genius that is Dan Haworth-Salter.

For the audiobook, blessings and salutations go to Alex Valentine for the studio space, engineering support, dry humour, and even drier cider. Double high-fives to James Kirk for the professional tech assistance, and Owen Carter for the game-changing lend of a superb microphone and other audio necessities.

To those who read early drafts and prodded me onwards, yet had no qualms about pointing out the terrible bits – now removed – thanks also. Honourable mentions here to Peter Wilkinson, Matthew Owen, Jessie White, Mark & Kaisa Phillips, and Emanation Smith for their early editing, highlighting, reading, and feedback.

Finally, to Layne Arlina – a woman who inspires me deeply with her strength and open-hearted approach to life. Who knew you were such a badass editorial genius? I'm eternally grateful for all the love and patience you have shown this project. It has been a blessing to spend this cycle with you.

This book is also dedicated to the memory of Chester, the most handsome and cuddly canine I have ever had the pleasure to know.

Supporting Chimera

It means a great deal to me that this story has finally been able to fly from the memory palace of my mind into the receptive eyes, ears and hearts of others.

If you enjoyed reading this book, please consider supporting its journey into the wider world by adding a review to the Good Reads website. You can find the listing here:

https://www.goodreads.com/book/show/59690268-chimera

Crowdfunder Supporters

This book was first launched via a crowdfunder campaign in August 2021. Backed by over 100 people, it raised just over £5K, enabling me to meet all my initial costs and donate £1K to various leukaemia and cancer charities.

I'd like to take the opportunity to thank each and every one of you early backers whose support for this project has been invaluable. You made all the difference.

The following names are presented in chronological order.

Dawn Fletcher

Steve & Sue White

Angie Francis

Matthew Hayman

Chris La Maison

Oliver Bettany

Adam Boon

Ian & Jo Pickering

Jason Schroeder

Jayne Worthington

David Morgan

Tamsin Fendley

Jane Thomas

Ben Mullard

Jessica Hamill

Carl Gent

Rose Bamford

Ian Baldwin

Emanation Smith

Ken Fisher

Simon Lewis

Maureen Ellis

Peter Wilkinson

Cyd Churchill

Gina Holsgrove

Kate Chesterton

Lucy Boyd

Alex Harvey

James Kirk

Ulrich Pickering

Justine Squire

Anna Cerrato

Richard Basgallop

Jessie White

AJ Leon

Stephen Carpenter

Anne-Marie Redhead

Josh White

Roger & Sarah Arguile

Rob Wear

Andreas Kornevall

Rose Hewlett

Lucy Fleetwood

Graham Bater

Michelle Goggi

Paul Stanyer

Jessica Eve Watkins

Rebecca Joy Card

James Rose

Lewis John

Martin Cooper

Ollie Gallant

Nicholas Bateman

Julie Burrows

Bethan Lloyd

Jim Brown

Jemma White

Gemma Whitelaw

Owen Carter

Ross Benzie

Willow Greenman

Chris & Sue White

Charles Anthony

Bea Martin

Claire Armstrong

Lee Kerr

Francesca Spickernell

Jonathan Smith

Nick Dodd

Russell Lewis

Owen Shiers

Jo Arnott

Matt & Laura Elliot

Bertie Playle

Olivia Preye-Bradbury

Kelvin Washbourn

Ross Macdougall

Tony Fan

Lula Edmonds

Jake Kirmes-Daly

Josh Humphries

Matthew Owen

Sophia Efthimiou

Molly Hopkins

Mark Reeves

Tess Ingleby

Annette Harrison

Jon Petherick

Mark & Kasia Phillips

Anna Dowdall

Spike Johnson

Kirsten Manley

Lucy Anderson

Emma Daman Thomas

Natasha Iwowo

Alice Clough

Sean Scullion

Judi Morgan

Vivienne Palmer-White

Mike Condon

Selena King

Angharad Wynne

Tommy Crawford

Layne Arlina

Paul Sammut

About the Author

Jody White was born in Wakefield, North Yorkshire, but grew up in the rural idyll of Bridgnorth, Shropshire.

An education in digital design took him east to Leicester, and later down to Brighton, East Sussex, where he spent over a decade forming strong friendships and absorbing the open-minded nature of alternative culture. On the south coast he fostered interests in shamanism, yoga, herbalism, and foraging, alongside his day job as a graphic designer, with evenings often spent playing drums with various bands.

In 2017, then living in St. Leonards-on-Sea, he founded *The Lumieres Podcast*, a slowly weaving thread of conversational interviews with figures who shine their light brightly in the world. Currently on hiatus, the podcast will resume in due course.

He currently lives in the Herefordshire Marches, a few miles from the border town of Y-Gelli / Hay-on-Wye.

Chimera is his first book.

To connect with Jody, use the following channels:

Personal website: www.jodywhite.co.uk
Facebook: @jodywhiteauthor
Instagram: @lifeinfractals
Podcast: www.lumierespodcast.com

Blood & Marrow

It would be remiss of me not to mention how important it is to consider registering on a bone marrow database, such as those operated by the British Bone Marrow Registry and The Anthony Nolan Trust. They link into a global network of registries. The more people signed up, the greater the chance of someone in need finding their match. You could literally save someone's life. If you are not currently part of a bone marrow register, please, I encourage you to take a few minutes out of your day when you can and sign up.

Likewise, if you've never given much thought to donating blood, I would urge you to contact your nearest hospital – or the NHS Blood & Transplant department – and ask them about the procedure. We are all made of this most sacred substance and clean blood is always in need in hospitals, especially if you have one of the rarer blood types. Please consider giving some of yours, feed the life of another human being.

British Bone Marrow Registry

https://www.bbmr.co.uk/

The Anthony Nolan Trust

https://www.anthonynolan.org/

NHS Blood & Transplant

https://www.nhsbt.nhs.uk/

This information is UK-centric, but blood donation is possible worldwide. Contact your local health centre and they should be able to point you in the right direction.